Workbook--Delivering Culturally Sensitive Nutrition Service$
—Responding to Clients' Iceberg Factors

by

Dr. Marcia Magnus

Marcia Magnus
magnus@fiu.edu
caramervoter@gmail.com

Printed in the United States of America

ISBN-10: 1-6505-9236-1
ISBN-13: 978-1650592367

Table of Contents

		Page
The Diet and Disease Link		4
Chapter 1	Quantifying the Cultural Sensitivity of Nutrition Service$	10
-		
Chapter 3	Targeting a Non-White Ethnic Group	21
Chapter 4	Securing Nutrition Co-Sponsors	27
Chapter 5	Preparing a Culturally Sensitive Nutrition Proposal	29
Chapter 6	The Continuum of XC Competence in Nutrition	41
Chapter 7	Culturally Sensitive Needs Assessment	47
Chapter 8	Culturally Sensitive Dietary Assessment	49
Chapter 9	Culturally Sensitive Nutrient Analysis	54
-		
Chapter 11	Ethnic Food Guide Pictorial Representations	61
Chapter 12	Culturally Sensitive Nutrition Counseling	67
Chapter 13	Culturally Sensitive Lesson Planning	71
Chapter 14	Culturally Sensitive Nutrition Program Planning	91
Chapter 15	Adapting Nutrition Education Materials	116
Chapter 16	Overcoming Dietary Obstacles	131
Making Oral Presentations		138

The Diet and Disease Link

DIETARY PRACTICES WHICH ARE POSITIVELY CORRELATED WITH CHRONIC DISEASES

Draw a line to link each chronic disease to dietary practices.

High Sugar Intake   Dental Caries

High Alcohol Intake   Cirrhosis

Excessive Salt Intake   Hypertension
                                       Stroke

Excessive Calorie Intake   Obesity
                                       Adult-Onset Diabetes

High Saturated Fat +
Cholesterol Intake   Coronary Heart Disease

Low Fiber Diet   Diverticulosis
                                       Constipation

High Fat Diet   Cancers:
                                       • Colon
                                       • Breast
                                       • Prostate

Low Calcium Diet   Osteoporosis

Dental caries or tooth _____ represents the number of missing, decayed or filled teeth. This is the only condition which has _____ in prevalence on this list. The addition of fluoride to the municipal _____ supply is responsible for the decline in the prevalence of dental caries. Too much fluoride causes fluorosis—the browning and mottling of teeth.

Cirrhosis of the liver represents the accumulation of fatty deposits in the liver due to extended _____ consumption. Cirrhosis is the precursor of _____ cancer. Alcohol consumption is _____ among college students than their non-college peers. A woman of the same height and weight as a man is _____ likely to become drunk because women have less alcohol dehydrogenase than men. Asian women have the smallest amount of alcohol dehydrogenase of all women.

If three women—a White, Black and Asian woman--of the same height and weight have 5 beers, who is more likely to get drunk first?

Hypertension represents elevated pressure of the blood throughout the arteries and veins. Approximately 33% of Americans have hypertension and the prevalence increases to 50% among _____ adults. The condition is asymptomatic for 90% of those afflicted, the remaining 10% suffer from dizziness or headaches. Many anti-hypertensive medications have the _____ effect of impotence (inability to sustain an erection). During the decade of the 20s, the _____ blood pressure level is 120/80mm of mercury. The non-dietary cure for hypertension is _____, and the dietary cure is high potassium intake approximately 5,000 mg.

Potassium-rich foods include:

Kale, frozen	1062 mg	1 cup
Collards, frozen	1059	1 cup
Spinach, frozen	1027	1 cup
Turnip greens, frozen	851	1 cup
Coconut water	500	1 cup (clear coconut water, not white cholesterol-raising coconut milk)
Orange juice	472	1 cup
Banana	467	1
Mustard greens	419	1 cup
Cucumber	301	1 large
Brussels sprouts	300	1 cup
Stewed prunes	248	1 cup

To meet daily potassium, a person would have to consume 10 bananas, and risk the possibility of having _____. However, to include green leafy vegetables at:

Breakfast:

Lunch:

Dinner:

Dessert:

The most important dietary recommendation for Americans is to eat five servings of fruits or vegetables every day to _____ the risk (likelihood of getting the condition) or delay the onset of multiple conditions—heart disease, hypertension, cancer, osteoporosis, diabetes, high blood cholesterol. The method of preparation of the fruits and vegetables is important. Fresh fruits have vitamin C, potassium, and fiber so they are nutritionally _____ to fruit juice, or cooked canned fruit in its own juice. Unsweetened dried fruit—raisins, prunes, apricots, and dates or _____ fruit are chock full of nutrients and they rarely _____. Sweetened dried fruit (cranberries, dried pineapple, kiwi, and mango) are recommended for those who wish to _____ weight.

Vegetables do not include starchy vegetables such as potatoes, and yuca. The most nutritious vegetables are _____ leafy vegetables. They are chockful of the anticancer vitamin A, vitamin C for cell renewal, and potassium which lowers blood _____. Fresh vegetables with low-fat dips such as hummus (chickpeas and ground sesame), and low-fat salad dressings are nutritionally _____ to regular salad dressing which is more than 70% fat calories.

Frozen vegetables will last for 6 months, but be sure to buy frozen vegetables which are 100% vegetable, with no additives. Creamed spinach is 66% _____ calories, while fresh spinach is 14% fat calories.

Stroke is the cessation of blood flow to the _____, causing physical, mental retardation and swallowing difficulties.

Obesity represents body weight which exceeds 20% of _____weight. Adult-onset diabetes represents uncontrolled blood sugar levels. Diabetes symptoms include excessive thirst, frequent urination, increased hunger and passing _____. Approximately 33% of White

American babies and 50% of non-White American babies who are born after the year 2000 will develop diabetes and have a shorter life expectancy than their _____.

Diabetes is abnormally high or low levels of blood sugar. Both hypogylcemia or low blood sugar and hyperglycemia or _____ blood sugar can result in passing out. The American Heart Association recommends that men have a maximum of 9 teaspoons of added sugar/day and 7 teaspoons/day for _____. Added sugar represents sugar which is not present in the natural food. Eight ounces of orange juice has 6 teaspoons of naturally occurring sugar. Apple sauce may have added sugar. A 6-ounce yogurt container has 7 teaspoons of added _____. The average American consumes 40 teaspoons every _____. A steady diet of excessive sugar and _____ leads to diabetes.

Coronary heart disease or a heart attack represents reduced blood flow to the heart muscle causing chest _____.

Diverticulosis is the formation of painful intestinal polyps. Diverticulitis is the inflammation of the polyps. Constipation, a common symptom of diverticulosis, is *painful*   *l* elimination of the feces, regardless of frequency. Excessive use of laxatives may lead to rectal prolapse.

Cancer of the colon represents an uncontrolled mushroom-shaped growth in the large bowel.

Breast cancer One of every eight women will develop breast cancer and the age of onset has been _____ in recent years. Women in their 30s and 40s are now being diagnosed. Foods which have aluminium wrappers; aluminium pots and aluminium in anti-perspirants contribute to

the development of Alzheimers' disease and tumor formation because aluminium is a heavy

_____ and a neurotoxin. Most breast tumors are found in the area of the _____

because the anti-perspirant blocks sweat formation, trapping the toxins inside the body.   For a

safer deodorizer, use _____ soda.

Prostate cancer represents the growth of the walnut-size gland just below the bladder.

Symptoms include difficulty starting to _____, increased frequency of urination,

nighttime bathroom trips for decreased force of volume of urine, leading to impotence, decreased

libido. Almost 80% of 80-year old men have prostate problems.

Osteoporosis represents_____ thinning where the bone tissue develops more and larger empty

spaces over time.

Chapter 1
Quantifying the Cultural Sensitivity of Nutrition Service$

Activity--<u>How Culturally Diverse Are Your Peers?</u>

1. If you or your parents were born in another country, please stand.

2. Name the country of your birth.

3. State an ethnic food that might be considered strange to others—the one that your Grandmother would be hesitant to share with a 25-year old registered dietitian nutritionist.

4. Describe its ingredients and how the food is prepared.

5. State one superfood of that culture. A superfood is high in an under consumed nutrient--fiber, omega-3 fats, magnesium, potassium, or vitamin A, or it may be low in an overconsumed nutrient—fat, sugar, or sodium.

Welcome to the "So You Want to Be a Vegan Workshop" at Whole Foods Market in Aventura, FL had

15 participants

- ☐ **3 Jamaicans**
- ☐ **2 Eastern Europeans**
- ☐ **3 African Americans**
- ☐ **4 Jewish Americans**
- ☐ **3 Whites**

The nutritionist shared samples and a recipe for a Vegan smoothie, along with samples dried beets. She described the nutritional strengths of each ingredient: almond milk, cocoa nibs, agave nectar, and ginseng.

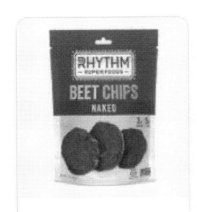 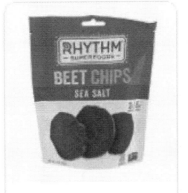

Among workshop participants, a member of each of the five ethnicities asked questions. Their ethnicities were obvious from their _____. They asked about the _____ of the beet chips, the best place to store cocoa nibs (fridge or countertop), and if chia seeds or flaxseed could be added to the smoothie. Each workshop participant received a Whole Foods Market reusable shopping bag, the weekly flyer, and a _____ for beet chips.

Unfortunately, the nutritionist made the mistake of Cultural Blindness—the assumption that we are all the same culturally, eating the same foods, and having the same food beliefs. She did not seize the opportunity to ask the Jamaican Americans, Russian Americans, African Americans, and White workshop participants to share their ethnic vegan _____. If she had asked the question:

"I'm hearing an accent, where are you _____?

What are some of your _____ vegan superfoods?"

They would have replied as follows:

Pumpkin soup, steamed callallo, a green leafy vegetable
Collard greens, black eye peas and rice
Hummus (ground chickpeas, sesame, garlic)
Oatmeal, blueberries, ground flaxseed
Borscht (beets and vegetable soup)

Match each of the following ethnicities with the ethnic vegan superfoods:

African Americans
Jamaican Americans
Jewish Americans
Whites
Russian Americans

If the nutritionist had asked about their individual accents and their superfoods, each workshop

participant would have _____ the workshop with multiple ethnic superfoods that they could add to

their vegan options. Instead, participants left the Vegan workshop without being able to _____

locally available ethnic vegan superfoods.

1. Identify the addresses, and meeting times of three local vegan groups--workshop, community
event, or Meetup group--that are close to your home or university zip code:
a.
b.
c.

2. Using your home or university zip code, state the names and addresses of three vegan
restaurants, include one Indian or Thai restaurant.
a.
b.
c.

Planning a Nutrition Program for the LGBT Community

To nutritionists, culturally different clients may belong to a specific ethnic group (Mexican, Venezuelan), a sports team where members are recruited from multiple countries, any sports teams (Basketball culture is different to the culture of jockeys), or the LGBT community.

The month of June was chosen for LGBT (lesbian, gay, bisexual, transgender) Pride Month to commemorate the Stonewall Inn police raid and riots in Greenwich Village, NYC, which occurred in June 1969. As a result, many pride events are held during this month to recognize the impact LGBT persons have had in the world.

LGBT Needs Assessment Data reveal that:

Approximately 10% of the US population describe themselves as homosexual. At the Gay Pride Parade, floats end in the area which includes: two mainstage areas for musicians, 120 community, booths, food and drink trucks, and family-friendly play areas. The 2018 Miami Gay Beach Pride welcomed a total of 145,000 persons.

-LGBT persons are also at higher risk of acquired immune deficiency syndrome AIDS and sexually transmitted diseases STDs than the general population.

-Lesbians and bisexual females are more likely to be overweight or obese than the general population.

-The nutritional mistakes of LGBT persons include:

Underconsumption of fruits, vegetables; magnesium, potassium, omega-3 fats, fiber.

Overconsumption of total fat, saturated fat, trans fat, sugar, alcohol.

Use the "Cross-Cultural Nutrition Checklist—Adapted for the LGBT Community" to plan nutrition programs for the LGBT community.

The Cross-Cultural Nutrition Checklist—Adapted for the LGBT Community

During the nutrition services...

1-Are the results of ethnic health/nutrition research shared?

2-Are visual success stories of LGBT clients shared?

3-Are health and nutrition issues among LGBT persons compared to the general population?

4-Are LGBT nutrition/health websites shared?

5-Is LGBT music used?

6-Are LGBT proverbs used?

7-Are LGBT celebrities and heroes used?

8-Are LGBT phrases and symbols used?

9-Are LGBT games and video games used to improve learning?

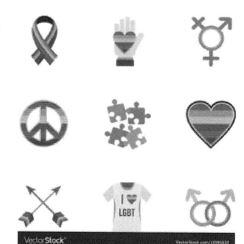

LGBT Nutrition Pride Month Program

It's January, six months before LGBT pride month, and your team of five students is developing a 1-page summary of LGBT Nutrition Pride Month Program as follows:

A. Develop titles for 3 nutrition tabling experiences for the 10-member Planning Committee of LGBT Pride Month:

i.

ii.

iii.

B. Prepare 5 low-budget nutritious refreshments for 3 meetings of the 10-member Planning Committee of LGBT Pride Month. List all the food and non-food items (tablecloths, napkins, plates, etc) that you will carry to each meeting:

Meeting 1

i. Food items--

Non food items--

Meeting 2

ii. Food items--

Non food items--

Meeting 3

iii. Food items--

Non food items--

C. Identify a named 20-minute nutrition activity for K-3rd grade children in the family-friendly area, specifying the grade level that you will target:

i.

D. Identify a 1-hour named nutrition activity for LGBT parents (childrens' food shopping or kitchen skills):

i.

E. Identify A 1-hour named LGBT youth nutrition activity for ages 12-18:

i.

Do You Need an Attitude Adjustment for this Exercise?

If this exercise makes you feel uncomfortable, this section is for you.

If you are afraid of, hate, feel uncomfortable around, or mistrust persons who are lesbian, gay, bisexual, or transgender, for the purposes of this activity,

please suspend your negative attitude.

Assume that a person who you love dearly has just told you that they are gay, and that you have decided that you will love them and all LGBT persons, no matter what.

Homophobia Scale

This questionnaire is designed to measure your thoughts, feelings, and behaviors with regards to homosexuality. It is not a test, so there are no right or wrong answers. Answer each item by circling the number after each question as follows:

1 Strongly agree
2 Agree
3 Neither agree nor disagree
4 Disagree
5 Strongly disagree

1. Gay people make me nervous.	1 2 3 4 5
2. Gay people deserve what they get.	1 2 3 4 5
3. Homosexuality is acceptable to me.	1 2 3 4 5
4. If I discovered a friend was gay I would end the friendship.	1 2 3 4 5
5. I think homosexual people should not work with children.	1 2 3 4 5
6. I make derogatory remarks about gay people.	1 2 3 4 5
7. I enjoy the company of gay people.	1 2 3 4 5
8. Marriage between homosexual individuals is acceptable.	1 2 3 4 5
9. I make derogatory remarks like "faggot" or "queer" to people I suspect are gay.	1 2 3 4 5
10. It does not matter to me whether my friends are gay or straight.	1 2 3 4 5
11. It would not upset me if I learned that a close friend was homosexual.	1 2 3 4 5
12. Homosexuality is immoral.	1 2 3 4 5
13. I tease and make jokes about gay people.	1 2 3 4 5
14. I feel that you cannot trust a person who is homosexual.	1 2 3 4 5
15. I fear homosexual persons will make sexual advances towards me.	1 2 3 4 5
16. Organizations which promote gay rights are necessary.	1 2 3 4 5
17. I have damaged property of gay persons, such as "keying" their cars.	1 2 3 4 5
18. I would feel comfortable having a gay roommate.	1 2 3 4 5
19. I would hit a homosexual for coming on to me.	1 2 3 4 5
20. Homosexual behavior should not be against the law.	1 2 3 4 5
21. I avoid gay individuals.	1 2 3 4 5
22. It does not bother me to see two homosexual people together in public.	1 2 3 4 5
23. When I see a gay person I think, "What a waste."	1 2 3 4 5
24. When I meet someone I try to find out if he/she is gay.	1 2 3 4 5
25. I have rocky relationships with people that I suspect are gay.	1 2 3 4 5

Source: http://www.midss.org/content/homophobia-scale

Scoring information for the Homophobia Scale (Wright, Adams, & Bernat)

1. Reverse score the following items: 1, 2, 4, 5, 6, 9, 12, 13, 14, 15, 17, 19, 21, 23, 24, 25 (to reverse score the items 1=5, 2=4, 3=3, 4=2, 5=1).

2. To calculate the total scale score, add items 1-25, then subtract 25 from the total scale score. The range of scores should then be between 0-100, with a score of 0 being the least homophobic and 100 being the most homophobic.

3. To calculate the subscale scores: (after items have been reverse scored)

    Factor 1 (Behavior/Negative Affect): add items 1, 2, 4, 5, 6, 7, 9, 10, 11, 22, then subtract 10. Scores should range between 0-40.

    Factor 2 (Affect/Behavioral Aggression): add items 12, 13, 14, 15, 17, 19, 21, 23, 24, 25, then subtract 10. Scores should range between 0-40.

    Factor 3 (Cognitive Negativism): add items 3, 8, 16, 18, 20, then subtract 5. Scores should range between 0-20.

Finding Checklist Features

The goal of this assignment is for you to estimate and then quantify the amount of time that it takes to find Checklist Features. You have decided to target the local Korean American Presbyterian Church for an 8-session nutrition program for two reasons. First, you discovered that Korean Americans are seven times more likely to be millionaires than non-Korean Americans. Second, you have always been curious about Koreans.

You are preparing a proposal for the church elders of a local Korean American church to fund your 8-session nutrition program.
1. Each student will estimate and write in the number of minutes to find the Checklist features.

2. Each student will set a timer to determine how many minutes and seconds it takes to find each Checklist feature.
One third of the class will estimate the first 4 Checklist features, the 3s.
One third of the class will estimate the second 4 Checklist features, the 2s.
One third of the class will estimate the last 5 Checklist features, the 1s.

3. Compare estimated and actual times to find Checklist features.

During the nutrition services…

	ESTIMATE	ACTUAL
3--Are ethnic food models used?		
3--Are the results of ethnic nutrition research shared?		
3--Are ethnic superfoods and nutritional strengths described?		
3--Are visual success stories of the clients' race shared?		
2--Are clients asked about their use of traditional healing systems?		
2--Is the health status of the ethnic group compared to Whites?		
2--Are ethnic nutrition websites shared?		
2--Do posters promote the use of interpreting services?		
1--Is ethnic music used?		
1--Are ethnic proverbs used?		
1--Are local heroes used?		
1--Are ethnic phrases and symbols used?		
1--Are ethnic games used?		

How accurate were your estimates?

<u>Video Assignment—HIV and Nutrition in the Male Community</u>

Watch the video and answer the following questions.

https://www.youtube.com/watch?v=O9dV8WdDGA0&t=182s

1. If you were a participant, would you return for the next session? Share your rationale in 2 lines.

2. Which 2 visuals would you add to the room to make it more appealing to the male gay community?

I would add visuals of...

1.

2.

3. Apply the LGBT Cross-Cultural Nutrition Checklist to the session. Using 1 line for each behavioral change, list 4 <u>behavioral</u> changes that you would make during the nutrition informational session. Define a specific behavior, not an attitude. "I would offer a handout which summarized the dietary recommendations" is a behavioral recommendation. "I would be more sensitive to their needs" is inappropriate because it is not a behavior.

I would...

A.

B.

C.

D.

Chapter 3
Targeting Non-White Populations for Nutrition Service$

Activity: Finding Multiple Community Groups of the Same Ethnicity

It's 2025, and you have completed a nutrition proposal for the largest local Mexican American church. List the names, addresses, and telephone numbers of five additional local Mexican American community groups to which you could adapt and pitch the nutrition proposal.

1.

2.

3.

4.

5.

<u>Checking your beliefs about an ethnic group</u>

To assess the importance of having a positive and negative attitude to an ethnic group, complete the following two activities.

Part 1

<u>Imagine Yourself Falling in Love with Your Ethnic Group</u>

1. Identify your favorite ethnic group and make a list of three attributes that you admire about this ethnic group. It could include their accent, ethnic superfoods, historical national triumphs, reputation, and customs (strong family ties).
Eg. Asian Americans are good with technology, value education, work hard, good in Math, they do not dwell on the past injustices, and they do not engage in civil unrest or protest.

Your ethnic group: _____
Their three admirable attributes: They are…
a.
b.
c.

2. Share the group's attributes with a classmate.

3. Respond to the question:
"How likely is it that your verbal and non-verbal communiques will be respectful and help you to bond with this ethnic group?" NOT THAT LIKELY/LIKELY/VERY LIKELY

Part 2

<u>Imagine Yourself Criticizing an Ethnic Group</u>

1.Make a list of three negative beliefs that you have about the **same** ethnic group. It could include the group's racial features, accent, ethnic red-light foods, historical events, negative stereotypes, and customs (minimum value on punctuality).
Eg. Asian Americans don't have any personality, they don't have good people skills, they are hard to connect with, they do not show emotions, and they are not fun to be around.

Your ethnic group:_____
Three negative beliefs about this group: They are…
a.
b.
c.

2. Share the group's attributes with a classmate.

3. Respond to the question: How likely is it that your verbal and non-verbal communiques will be respectful and bond with this ethnic group? NOT THAT LIKELY/LIKELY/VERY LIKELY

4. Share one insight with your classmate that you gained from taking these two perspectives of intentionally falling in love, and falling out of love with the same ethnic group.

HOW TO MODIFY A RECIPE

Insert the correct word at each _____.

If your recipe calls for this ingredient:	Substitute this ingredient for a heart-healthy alternative:
Bacon	_____ bacon, turkey bacon, smoked turkey or lean prosciutto (Italian ham)
Bread, white	Whole-grain bread
Bread crumbs, dry	Blended rolled _____ into a powder or crushed bran cereal
Butter, margarine, shortening or oil in baked goods	Applesauce or prune puree for half of the called-for butter, shortening or oil; butter spreads or shortenings specially formulated for baking that don't have trans fats Note: To avoid dense, soggy or flat baked goods, don't substitute oil for butter or shortening. Also don't substitute diet, whipped or tub-style margarine for regular margarine.
Butter, margarine, shortening or oil to prevent sticking	Cooking spray or nonstick pans
Cream	Fat-free half-and-half, evaporated _____ milk
Cream cheese, full fat	Fat-free or low-fat cream cheese, Neufchatel, or low-fat cottage cheese pureed until smooth
Eggs	Two egg whites or 1/4 cup egg substitute for each whole egg
Flour, all-purpose (plain)	Whole-wheat flour for half of the called-for all-purpose flour in baked goods Note: Whole-wheat pastry flour is less dense and works well in softer products like cakes and muffins.
Fruit canned in heavy syrup	Fruit canned in its _____ juices or in water, or fresh fruit
Ground beef	Extra-lean or lean ground beef, chicken or turkey breast (make sure no poultry skin has been added to the product)
Lettuce, iceberg	Arugula, chicory, collard greens, dandelion greens, kale, mustard greens, spinach or watercress
Mayonnaise	Reduced-calorie mayonnaise-type salad dressing or reduced-calorie, reduced-fat mayonnaise
Meat as the main ingredient	Three times as much vegetables as the meat on pizzas or in casseroles, soups and stews
Milk, evaporated	Evaporated skim milk
Milk, whole	Reduced-fat or fat-free milk
Oil-based marinades	Wine, balsamic vinegar, fruit juice or fat-free broth
Pasta, enriched (white)	_____ wheat pasta
Rice, white	Brown rice, wild rice, bulgur or pearl barley
Salad dressing	Fat-free or reduced-calorie dressing or flavored vinegars
Seasoning salt, such as garlic salt, celery salt or onion salt	Herb-only seasonings, such as garlic powder, celery seed or onion flakes, or use finely chopped herbs or garlic, celery or onions

Soups, creamed	Fat-free milk-based soups, mashed potato flakes, or pureed carrots, potatoes or tofu for thickening agents
Soups, sauces, dressings, crackers, or canned meat, fish or vegetables	Low-sodium or reduced-sodium versions
Sour cream, full fat	Fat-free or low-fat sour cream, plain fat-free or low-fat yogurt
Soy sauce	Sweet-and-sour sauce, hot mustard sauce or low-sodium soy sauce
Sugar	In most baked goods you can reduce the amount of sugar by one-half; intensify sweetness by adding vanilla, nutmeg or _____
Syrup	Pureed fruit, such as applesauce, or low-calorie, sugar-free syrup
Table salt	Herbs, spices, citrus juices (lemon, lime, orange), rice vinegar, salt-free seasoning mixes or herb blends
Yogurt, fruit-flavored	Plain yogurt with fresh fruit slices
Bacon	Canadian bacon, turkey bacon, smoked turkey or lean prosciutto (Italian ham)
Bread, white	Whole-grain bread
Bread crumbs, dry	Rolled oats or crushed bran cereal
Butter, margarine, shortening or oil in baked goods	Applesauce or prune puree for half of the called-for butter, shortening or oil; butter spreads or shortenings specially formulated for baking that don't have trans fats Note: To avoid dense, soggy or flat baked goods, don't substitute oil for butter or shortening. Also don't substitute diet, whipped or tub-style margarine for regular margarine.
Butter, margarine, shortening or oil to prevent sticking	Cooking spray or nonstick pans
Cream	Fat-free half-and-half, evaporated skim milk
Cream cheese, full fat	Fat-free or low-fat cream cheese, Neufchatel, or low-fat cottage cheese pureed until smooth
Eggs	Two egg whites or 1/4 cup egg substitute for each whole egg
Flour, all-purpose (plain)	Whole-wheat flour for half of the called-for all-purpose flour in baked goods Note: Whole-wheat pastry flour is less dense and works well in softer products like cakes and muffins.
Fruit canned in heavy syrup	Fruit canned in its own juices or in water, frozen or _____ fruit
Ground beef	Extra-lean or lean ground beef, chicken or turkey breast (make sure no poultry skin has been added to the product)
Lettuce, iceberg	Arugula, chicory, collard greens, dandelion greens, kale, mustard greens, spinach or watercress
Mayonnaise	Reduced-calorie mayonnaise-type salad dressing or reduced-calorie, reduced-fat mayonnaise
Meat as the main ingredient	Three times as many vegetables as the meat on pizzas or in casseroles, soups and stews
Milk, evaporated	Evaporated skim milk

Milk, whole	Reduced-fat or fat-free milk
Oil-based marinades	Wine, balsamic vinegar, fruit juice or fat-free broth
Pasta, enriched (white)	Whole-wheat pasta
Rice, white	Brown rice, wild rice, bulgur or pearl barley
Salad dressing	Fat-free or reduced-calorie dressing or flavored vinegars
Seasoning salt, such as garlic salt, celery salt or onion salt	Herb-only seasonings, such as garlic powder, celery seed or onion flakes, or use finely chopped herbs or garlic, celery or onions
Soups, creamed	Fat-free milk-based soups, mashed potato flakes, or pureed carrots, potatoes or tofu for thickening agents
Soups, sauces, dressings, crackers, or canned meat, fish or vegetables	Low-sodium or reduced-sodium versions
Sour cream, full fat	Fat-free or low-fat sour cream, plain fat-free or low-fat yogurt
Soy sauce	Sweet-and-sour sauce, hot mustard sauce, or low-_____ soy sauce
Sugar	In most baked goods you can reduce the amount of sugar by one-half; intensify sweetness by adding vanilla, nutmeg or cinnamon
Syrup	Pureed fruit, such as applesauce, or low-calorie, sugar-free syrup
Table salt	Herbs, spices, citrus juices (lemon, lime, orange), rice vinegar, salt-free seasoning mixes or herb blends
Yogurt, fruit-flavored	Plain yogurt with fresh fruit slices, or frozen fruit

Chapter 4
Securing A Nutrition Co-Sponsor

Activity—Identifying potential co-sponsors

a. Think of a city that you would like to live in.

Identify the county where the county is located.

Review the most recent data on:

1. the top largest companies, by revenue
2. the top largest companies, by number of employees
3. the most diverse companies in your home zip code

List the 2 largest companies and their annual revenue:

a.

b.

List the 2 largest companies and number of employees:

a.

b.

Identify the 5 most diverse companies in your home zip code. Underline the companies that you have ever patronized. Having patronized those companies, you are now in a position to describe your history with the company during your request for co-sponsorship of your nutrition program. The 5 most diverse companies in my zip code are:

a.

b.

c.

d.

e.

Activity--Being SUAVE in your communications:
1. Form a group of 2 students.
2. The shorter student will be interviewed. For this activity, the shorter student needs to assume a new name.
3. The taller student will be the interviewer. Ask the shorter student to share their name.
4. For 2 minutes, the taller student will ask the following questions, using the

SUAVE guidelines:
a. Ask about the spelling of the person's name,
b. Make an association of the person's name with something strange but memorable. If the interviewee's name is Suarez, the association to remember the name Suarez would be: sue a reservation.
c. Use the person's name (Senora Suarez) in every other question.
d. End the conversation by using the person's name.

while asking the following questions:
-Hello, I am _____. Tell me your name. How do you spell that?
-One of the best ways to determine diet quality is to assess fruit and vegetable intake. How many fruits and vegetables did you have yesterday?
-Did you add anything to the fruits?
-Did you add anything to the vegetables?
-What made it hard for you to have the 5 recommended servings?
-How many fruits and vegetables you think you'll have tomorrow?

4. Switch roles--Shorter person is the interviewer
-Hello, I am _____. Tell me your name. How do you spell that?
-One of the best ways to determine diet quality is to assess fruit and vegetable intake. How many fruits and vegetables did you have yesterday?
-Did you add anything to the fruits?
-Did you add anything to the vegetables?
-What made it hard for you to have the 5 recommended servings?
-How many fruits and vegetables you think you'll have tomorrow?

After Action Report:
How many people heard their name
Once?
2 times?
3 times?
4 times?
5 times?

What was the hardest part of using the SUAVE guidelines?

Chapter 5

Preparing A Culturally Sensitive Nutrition Proposal

Which Nutrition Positions Need to Use Culturally Sensitive Strategies?

Among the following positions which require a bachelor's degree in Nutrition but not an RD credential, which do not require the use of Checklist features--ethnic health disparities, proverbs, music, phrases, symbols?

- Quality control supervisor for a food processing plant
- Public health inspector (of restaurants)
- Food service equipment specialist
- Restaurant owner or manager
- Chef--restaurant, retirement community, school, cruise ship programming for passengers)
- Caterer for events, daily meal service, congregate meals
- Restaurant consultant for food labeling or menu analysis
- Community nutrition educator--university, worksite wellness program
- Cooking demonstrator or Culinary educator
- Non-profit organization nutritionist such as WIC
- Nutrition educator, health-related organizations--American Heart/Diabetes/Obesity Association
- Team leader for organizations--Common Threads, Flipany, Feed My Starving Children
- Nutrition educator--weight loss camp, juvenile summer diabetes camp
- Dietary supervisor
- Consumer communications with a food company
- Program director for a government education program
- Food scientist
- Food service administrator
- Food service manager
- Health food store management
- Sales representative for supplement, medical, aesthetic, or pharmaceutical company
- Grant writer
- Marketing specialist for food companies, nutrition publications, or organizations
- Public relations for food companies, nutrition publications, or organizations
- Website developer for nutrition professionals
- Brand ambassador for food-related companies
- Nutrition writer for health newsletter, magazine, blog, online forum
- Social media writer for companies
- Nutrition coach, Wellness coach
- Author
- 4-H Extension service
- Food advertising consultant
- Food photography specialist
- Food research and marketing specialist
- Food stylist (creates and photographs foods on menus, articles)

If people are buying food there or eating there, there is an opportunity for you to add value by reversing their nutrition problems!

Non-Verbal Communication with Specific Cultural Groups

Fill in the blanks for the following guidelines.

There are distinct cultural differences in non-verbal behavior across non-White groups. In this context, non-Whites include those who are Hispanic of all races, multiethnic Black Americans, multiethnic Asian and Pacific Islanders, Native Americans, and _____ Americans of all ethnicities such as Lebanese, Egyptians, and Syrians. Culturally sensitive nutrition professionals use culturally appropriate gesturing and body movements, facial expressions, eye contact, touch, and seating arrangements to develop rapport (Klement, 2010). Some cultures value closeness and warmth, while others perceive distance as an indication of respect and high regard. To ignore culture-specific non-verbal communication norms is to enlarge the disconnect between nutritionist and culturally different clients. One of the reasons why culturally different clients prefer health care professionals who share their ethnicity is because the professionals know, respect, and use culture-specific verbal and non-verbal communication _____.

The following guidelines are recommended for communicating non-verbally with specific cultural groups. They are not intended to stereotype or suggest that _____ members in the ethnic group adhere to the same beliefs.

For the following sections, read the section and then choose between the ethnic group separated by a "/" in the title:

Mexican/Asian Americans – Feel they are punctual even if they are 20 minutes late and view tardiness as a sign of respect. They shake hands forcefully and for longer periods of time, and may want to engage in extensive small talk before opening u p . Asking them about their interests and <u>families</u> before beginning the session will create trust. The counselor will be viewed as an authority figure and will be expected to dress professionally. Once trust has been established, they are likely to form a close bond. Interrupting the speaker is not considered impolite. Although they <u>converse at close ranges</u> and signs of <u>affection</u> are encouraged, they are uncomfortable with extended eye contact.
If complimenting a child, <u>touch</u> them briefly, otherwise it may cause <u>evil eye</u> in the c l i e n t 's belief system. They may not accept the invitation to ask questions until offered two or three times to do so. The soles of the feet or bottom of the shoe should not be shown, as it is perceived as being rude to do so. The "OK" sign in the United States (made using the thumb and index finger) is an obscene gesture. The husband is responsible for making health decisions and should be included in the counseling session.

African/Asian Americans – Converse at close range and use significant amounts of hand gesturing when speaking. They maintain continuous eye contact while speaking, but broken eye contact while listening. They prefer indirect questions and equal turn taking during conversations. They believe it is appropriate to interrupt another. Touching the top of the head is a personal violation. They may feel a first name basis infers disrespect, especially with elder patients, and prefer to be greeted by last name and respective title: Mr., Mrs., Ms. or Miss. Decisions regarding health issues will be viewed as a family responsibility. The head of the household, which is typically the female, should be involved in decision making.

White Northerners/Native Americans – Family takes precedence over an individual. Values include sharing, cooperation, and spirituality. Being a collective group with a present time orientation can make them late for a health appointment. In greeting, a smile and handshake are customary, although a vigorous handshake may be perceived as an aggressive act. Elders are highly respected, and should be referred to as "grandmother" or "grandfather" in conversation. They may want to engage in extensive small talk before opening up, and may believe the health professional should be able to deduce the problem through instinct. Their personal space is greater than Hispanic cultures, and they will shun eye contact as a symbol of respect. Nodding their head indicates they are listening but does not suggest an understanding of the message or that they are in agreement with what is being said. As it is deemed impolite to take notes, ask them to repeat what they have understood during the conversation. Clients speak for themselves and expect an unhurried conversation that is informal and interactive. They use silence as a sign of respect and believe that if they speak too quickly before silently contemplating their answer, they may be viewed as being immature. Being comfortable with silence, they may take 90 seconds or more to respond to a question. The professional should speak in a normal volume, because loudness is considered disrespectful, as is pointing with the hands. "Yes" or "no" can be the complete answer to a question. If they do not wish to discuss a matter, they may say they "don't know."

Caribbean/Chinese Americans – They may arrive late to the meeting without apology. The first word in their name is family name, the second word is their middle name, and the last one or two words are their given name. They usually prefer being addressed by their family name along with Mr. or Mrs., but the health professional should ask the client how they would like to be addressed. Upon greeting, they may not smile but rather nod their head or bow slightly. Handshaking may or may not be appropriate so it is best to wait for an extended hand. Touching is uncommon.

In conversation settings, they prefer to sit next to someone vs. across the desk or table. Less personal space is preferred, sitting and standing closer to the counselor albeit avoiding eye contact. They may want to engage in extensive small talk before opening up. Nodding of the head indicates they are listening but does not suggest an understanding of the message or that they agree. Ask them to repeat the information. Silence is a form of respect, and it is best not to interrupt their process. They will also need the health professional to maintain a positive outlook on the results of following their treatment plan. They may need to be asked several times if they do not understand something. When the nutrition professional asks questions, to <u>save face</u> the client may say "yes" to avoid any confrontation, even if their answer is "no."

Gesturing with hands while talking may make them feel uncomfortable. Pointing with the index finger is regarded as ill-mannered. <u>Expressing emotion is regarded as immature.</u> However, if they are uncomfortable or surprised, they may noisily suck in air to express their negative emotion. Seldom will they publicly <u>show physical contact,</u> and touching the top of their head is a violation. The soles of the feet or shoes should not be shown as it is perceived as being arrogant and rude. Crossing the legs in considered inappropriate. Good posture is important to them.

African/Filipino Americans– Men may find discomfort working with a female health figure and will refrain from maintaining prolonged eye contact. T o avoid conflict and <u>save face, emotions are pent up</u> and the patient will appear polite and cooperative. They are sensitive to social slights so preventing embarrassment in the meeting is paramount. Giggling or smiling can indicate discomfort or interest. They are comfortable with silence and require a greater personal space. The use of first names should be avoided when greeting adults who are older. The middle name is the mother's maiden name, and the last name is the father's name.

African/Vietnamese Americans- May arrive late to their appointment. By avoiding direct eye contact, they are indicating respect. They will require more personal space than other cultures. The family name is written first, the middle name is next, with the first name listed last. They usually prefer their first name along with Mr. or Mrs. A patriarchal culture, men will not be accustomed to working with women in the health care setting. Men will shake hands, but it is respectful to wait for a <u>woman to offer her hand first.</u> Expressing their emotions and feelings is not something they are accustomed to doing and consider it a weakness that interferes with self-control. Negative emotions may be expressed by silence. To avoid conflict, smiling is a common reaction. Explain the program as accurately and as simply as possible and ask them to repeat what they've understood. Nodding of the head does not necessarily indicate approval or understanding. The <u>head is considered sacred</u> and must not be touched. Feet, being the lowest part of the body, are offensive and should not be shown.

African/Korean Americans – Direct eye contact demonstrates sincerity and is expected. T h e y d o <u>n o t s h o w emotions</u>, and appear cold and distant. Too much smiling is viewed as the mark of a superficial person. Very <u>little touching</u> occurs in public, although a light introductory handshake is typical. When rising to shake hands in greeting an elder, it is customary to <u>touch the palm of the left hand to the elbow of the right arm</u>. This gesture is also traditionally employed in passing items. In seating arrangements, the seat to the right is regarded as one of honor. Crossing legs is taboo. They view <u>loudness or laughing as impolite</u>. They are hesitant to say "no," but will indicate disagreement by tipping the head and sucking air in through their teeth. The

"OK" sign using the thumb and index finger in the United States indicates money to Koreans.

Arab/South Americans –They come from any one of 21 states or countries where the same language is spoken. In 2010, foreign-born persons were from:
Lebanese: 485,917
Egyptian: 179,853
Syrian: 147,426
Palestinian: 83,241
Moroccan: 74,908
Iraqi: 73,896
Jordanian: 60,056
Yemeni 29,358 (Michigan State School of Journalism, 2019).

Arab Americans may run up to 30-60 minutes late for an appointment. At the beginning and end of each visit, shake hands less firmly but longer than usual. However, do not touch members of the opposite sex or extend a hand to an Arab female unless she initiates the handshake. Smile and greet in order of seniority, but males are always greeted first. They prefer to be addressed using a title and their first name. Eye contact is important and is long in duration. They may resist the pressure to achieve too much at the first meeting and will want to spend time with small talk before opening up. The counselor can gain trust by sharing a bit of personal information with them. Coffee or tea should be offered at least three times. The appointment should remain unhurried. Looking at your watch suggests they are not worthy of your time. They use direct body orientation when engaged in conversation and are communicative, animated, and speak with volume to denote strength. Responding with silence in conversation is viewed as negative, while interrupting the speaker is not considered impolite. Nodding the head indicates they are listening but does not suggest an understanding of the message or that they are in agreement.

Refrain from bright colors in dress, and avoid cologne or perfume, as they believe a person's bodily smell is important. Do not pass objects with the left hand as it is considered unclean. Good posture when standing and sitting shows respect and proper manners. When the "OK" sign is accompanied by exposing teeth, it indicates hostility. Showing the bottom of the foot or pointing with the index finger is considered rude. The Arab client may not actively take part in decision-making, but see their role as cooperating with the program that has been outlined for them.

White/Japanese Americans – They are "fashionably late" to events. In order to demonstrate respect, they should not be addressed on a first-name basis. A light handshake is customary. They prefer an unhurried meeting and may want to engage in long periods of conversation before getting to the agenda of their appointment. Silence is used when considering something and also can indicate respect, rather than a lack of desire to continue the conversation. Criticism leads to embarrassment and a halt in the communication flow. Waving a hand with palm facing outward in front of the face signals "I don't know." They may inhale breath to signal respect while communicating with others. They do not verbalize emotion and may hide anger or sorrow by smiling and laughing. <u>Displays of emotion are considered rude</u> and lacking in control. Physical contact is not likely to be shown in public. <u>Downcast or closed eyes indicate attentiveness</u> and agreement. Direct eye contact is regarded as discourteous, intimidating, and disrespectful. They feel uncomfortable when people gesture with their hands while speaking. Even the slightest gesture could have meaning and therefore it is best to refrain from hand or body gestures. They <u>relate status and authority to dress</u> more than anywhere else in the world. Good posture is highly regarded.

Asian Indians/African Americans – In greeting, acknowledge the husband first. He may also be the <u>spokesperson for his wife</u>. Very little physical contact is shown although a handshake may work. They will be soft-spoken, courteous, and polite. Asian Indian women will not be comfortable with male counselors and will not maintain eye contact. Direct eye contact between women and men is avoided for reasons of modesty and religious laws. However, men may engage in direct eye contact and will be highly respectful of health professionals. They will not expect to be rushed in the meeting and will engage in significant small talk. The meeting should be leisurely or they will perceive the practitioner as rude. It is impolite to point with the <u>foot as it is regarded as the filthiest part of the body.</u> Do not cross the leg and show the bottom of the foot. Touching the head should be avoided, as well as any sign of affection or touching. The <u>left hand is considered unclean.</u>

Adapted from:

Klement C. *Intercultural Competence for the Nutrition Professional.* 2010. Thesis. Eastern Michigan University http://commons.emich.edu/cgi/viewcontent.cgi?article=1212&context=honors. Accessed May 27, 2019.

Michigan State School of Journalism. https://news.jrn.msu.edu/culturalcompetence/ethnicity/arab-americans/#ancestry. April 23, 2019.

Bias Busters: Cultural competence guides on race, religion and more Accessed June 29,2019.

Activity—Marketing a Beauty Shop Weight Loss Program

You are planning a Weight Loss program for Puerto Rican beauty shop. For each of the following obstacles to program participation, identify one strategy which could be incorporated into the flyer development and marketing.

OBSTACLE   STRATEGY
1.No time to come
2.I know what I need to eat
3.I'm eating okay
4.I'd be embarrassed
5.Child care

List 10 ways to market the program to Puerto Rican beauty shop patrons.

1.   6.
2.   7.
3.   8.
4.   9.
5.   10.

List 10 ways to advertise the weight loss program in a Puerto Rican American church:

1.   6.
2.   7.
3.   8.
4.   9.
5.   10.

Calculating Daily % Plant Protein

To conduct a 24-hour food recall,

1. Enter the portion size of each food and beverage consumed into a nutrient database (myfitnesspal.com)

2. Enter each ingredient in combination foods. For Mexican menudo, include tripe, onion, garlic, oregano, rosemary, guajillo sauce, beef stock, hominy corn, potatoes

3. Star the animal foods and beverages that were consumed—any dairy, seafood, meat, eggs.

4. Add the number of grams of animal protein in each animal food or beverage to get the total animal protein intake.

5. From the printout, get the total number grams of protein consumed.

6. % plant protein= plant protein/total protein * 100

% animal protein= 100 -% plant protein

24-Hour Food Recall—Juan Perez

	Animal Protein (calculated)	Total Protein (from printout)
Breakfast: none		
Lunch:		
-Churros 5 pieces	0	4
-16 oz Coke	-	-
-2 steak burritos	28*	42
Dinner: Jack-In-The-Box		
-2 chicken chimichangas	40**	48
-1 Mandarin Jarritos soda 25oz	-	-
-Menudo 1 cup	27***	30
Total protein	95 animal PRO	124 plant PRO

% animal protein=
% plant protein =
AHA recommendation 67% plant protein, 33% animal

*Amount of Animal Protein in 2 steak burritos?
Steak burrito ingredients--https://www.caciqueinc.com/blog/skirt-steak-tacos-with-cotija-cheese/

- 1 pound lean skirt steak
- 2 tablespoons of your favorite meat rub
- 12 small 6 inch tortillas
- 1 cup crumbled Cacique® Cotija Cheese
- 1 avocado peeled and sliced
- 3/4 cup fresh cilantro chopped
- Fresh salsa
- 1 whole avocado
- 2/3 cup Cacique® Crema Mexicana
- 1/2 cup fresh cilantro
- 1/4 teaspoon garlic powder
- Salt and Pepper to taste   Serves 12 tortillas

Animal foods in steak burrito=lean flank steak, Cacique® Cotija Cheese, Cacique® Crema Mexicana
Client had 2 tortillas.
16 oz lean flank steak serves 12 tortillas.
Client had 2 tortillas or 16/6 of steak=2.67 oz
3 oz flank steak has 24.4 g protein-- https://www.menshealth.com/nutrition/a19527826/flank-steak-nutrition-facts/
2.67 oz flank steak has 21.7g protein
1 cup Cacique® Cotija Cheese=0g protein

2/3 cup Cacique® Crema Mexicana=0g protein

Total animal protein in 2 steak burritos=21.7g

Amount of Animal protein in 2 Chicken chimichangas (Jack-In-The-Box)?
Chimichanga Ingredients-- https://www.fatsecret.com/calories-nutrition/generic/chimichanga-with-chicken-and-cheese

53 g Flour tortillas

40 g Chicken meat (broilers or fryers, stewed)

16 g Iceberg lettuce (includes crisphead types)

22 g Radishes

32 g Cheddar cheese

21 g Vegetable oil (industrial, partially hydrogenated soy, non-dairy butter flavor)

0.3 g Salt

Animal protein sources in chicken chimichanga are chicken and cheese.
Grams of protein from chicken:
40 g chicken=1.4 oz.
Chicken meat, cooked (4 ounces): 35 grams protein
1.4 oz chicken=(1.4/4) x 35=.35 x 35=12.25g chicken (animal) protein
Grams of protein from cheese:
32 g cheddar cheese=1.13 oz.
1 oz. cheddar cheese= 7 grams protein
1.13 oz cheese=1.13 x 7=7.91 grams cheese (animal) protein
Total number of animal protein grams in 1 chicken chimichanga=
12.25 g (chicken) + 7.91 g (cheese) =20.16g

***Amount of Animal Protein in Menudo?

Menudo Ingredients--https://www.mylatinatable.com/authentic-mexican-menudo-recipe/

- 2 Pounds of Rumba Meats Honeycomb Tripe
- 1 Liter of Water
- ½ White Onion
- 1 head of garlic about 4-5 cloves
- 1 Branch of Fresh Oregano
- 1 Branch of Fresh Rosemary
- ½ teaspoon of Salt
- Guajillo Sauce 2 pasilla peppers, 2 guajillo peppers, salt, pepper, cumin, clove of garlic
- 1 Can of Beef Stock
- 1 Can of Hominy
- 2 Potatoes cut into medium sized cubes

Recipe had 4 servings

2 pounds tripe=32 oz

Client had 1 serving

1 serving =32/4=8oz

3 oz tripe has 10 g animal protein--https://www.livestrong.com/article/470909-is-tripe-good-for-you/

Client therefore had 8/3=2.7 x 10=27g animal protein in 1 8 oz. serving of menudo

Chapter 6
The Continuum of Cross-Cultural Competence in Nutrition

<u>Finding Ethnic Nutrition Websites</u>

You are counseling an African American, Mexican American and Chinese American client who is overweight and has been diagnosed with diabetes. Identify one website that you would recommend for each client. For each website, in 2 lines, 12 font, describe one feature that you would change as you present the website to the client.

1. African American client:

2. Hispanic American client:

3. Asian American client:

Improving the FDPIR

The common health problems of Native Americans include:
higher rates of overweight, obesity, diabetes, amputations, hypercholesterolemia, hypertension, and cancer than non-Native groups.

The common nutritional mistakes among Native Americans include:
underconsumption of fruits, vegetables, legumes; potassium, plant protein, fiber, magnesium, and omega-3 fats; and overconsumption of total fat, saturated fat, white flour, sugar, and sodium.

List of Food Distribution Program for Indian Reservation Foods

(Highlighted data added to facilitate interpretation of diet quality)

Fruits	Teaspoons sugar/cup
A. Grape juice, Concord, 100% unsweetened	7
Cranberry apple juice, 100% unsweetened	7
Apple juice, 100% unsweetened	6
Cherry apple juice, 100% unsweetened	6
Applesauce, unsweetened	5
Orange juice, 100% unsweetened	5

B. Fruit and nut mix, dried--62% fat calories

C. Apricots, halves, extra light syrup, canned
Mixed fruit, extra light syrup, canned
Peaches, sliced, extra light syrup, canned
Pears, extra light syrup, canned
Cranberries, dried

D. Plums, pitted, dried
Raisins, unsweetened
Blueberries, frozen

Protein foods	Protein calories
-Tuna chunk light, canned	88%
-Beef, canned 5g fat x 9= 45/110=41% fat calories; 17 g protein x 4=68/110=	62%
-Chicken, canned 20% fat calories,	80%
-Chicken, boneless breast, frozen, 5% fat calories,	75%
-Chicken, whole, frozen 38% fat calories,	60%
-Beef, round roast, frozen 36% fat calories,	60%
-Pork loin chops, boneless, frozen 43% fat calories,	51%
-Beef stew, canned 48% fat calories,	48%

The following "protein" foods are higher in % _____ calories than % protein calories:
-Beef, fine ground, 85% lean, 15% fat, frozen--63% fat calories,   35% protein calories
(4 oz 85% lean ground beef has 17 grams of fat;1 gram of fat has 9 calories:
17 x 9=153/243=63% fat calories)
-Egg mix, dried 65% fat,   24% protein calories
-Peanut butter, smooth 71% fat calories,   19% protein calories
-Peanuts, roasted, unsalted 78% fat calories,   18% protein calories

Vegetables
Beans, green, low-sodium, canned
Carrots, sliced, low-sodium, canned
Corn, whole kernel, no salt added, canned
Hominy, low-sodium, canned
Mixed vegetables, 7-way blend, canned
Peas, green, low-sodium, canned
Potatoes, dehydrated flakes
Potatoes, sliced, low-sodium
Spaghetti sauce, low-sodium
Spinach, low-sodium, canned
Tomato juice, low-sodium
Tomato sauce, low-sodium
Tomato soup, condensed, low-sodium
Vegetable soup condensed, low-sodium, canned

Tomatoes, diced, no salt added
Peas, green, frozen

Legumes
Beans, black, low-sodium, canned
Beans, kidney, light red, low-sodium, canned
Beans, pinto, low-sodium, canned
Beans, refried, low-sodium, canned
Beans, vegetarian, low-sodium, canned

Beans, pinto, dry
Beans, Great Northern, dry

How do you rate the likelihood of these 2020 FDPIR foods to correct nutritional mistakes and improve the nutritional status of Native Americans?
A. VERY GOOD
B. GOOD
C. NOT THAT GOOD

Among the 2020 FDPIR foods, four overconsumed nutrients include:
a.
b.
c.
d.

Five under consumed nutrients in the 2020 FDPIR foods include:

a.

b.

c.

d.

e.

American Academy of _____ --Recommendations on Fruit Juice, 2017

--Infants (up to 12 months) should not be given fruit juice.
--Intake of juice should be limited to, at most, 4 ounces daily for toddlers age 1-3.
--For children age 4-6, fruit juice should be restricted to 4 to 6 ounces daily.
--For children ages 7-18, juice intake should be limited to 8 ounces or 1 cup of the recommended 2 to 2 ½ cups of fruit servings per day.
--Toddlers should not be given juice from bottles or easily transportable "sippy cups" that allow them to consume juice easily throughout the day. The excessive exposure of the teeth to carbohydrates can lead to tooth decay, as well. Toddlers should not be given juice at bedtime.
--Children should be encouraged to eat whole fruits and be educated about the benefits of the fruit as compared with juice, which lacks dietary fiber and may contribute to excessive weight gain.

American Academy of _____. American Academy of _____ Recommends No Fruit Juice for Children Under 1 Year. https://www.aap.org/en-us/about-the-aap/aap-press-room/Pages/American-Academy-of-.........................-Recommends-No-Fruit-Juice-For-Children-Under-1-Year.aspx 2017.

Activity—Creating heart-healthy dishes from FDPIR foods
Review the FDPIR food list in Chapter 6. Create 5 heart-healthy dishes for BLDS by using existing FDPIR foods. Chili—beans, ground beef, canned tomato.
1.omelet with
2.lasagna with
3.smoothie with
4.soup with
5.casserole with

*You have secured a consultancy with the USDA. Your role is to assess the program and make recommendations which will NOT increase **shipping costs**. Based on their current disease profile, list 9 foods which, if included in the FDPIR food package, could improve the nutritional status of Native Americans?*

1.   *6.*

2.   *7.*

3.   *8.*

4.   *9.*

5.

Canned foods may increase the risk of leptospirosis--nausea and vomiting which can be fatal in those who have auto-immune disorders (lupus, HIV/AIDS, and rheumatoid arthritis). Persons who use canned foods need to wash all cans with hot, soapy water to reduce the risk of leptospirosis from dehydrated rat urine in warehouses. A warning notice among the canned foods would alert Native American FDPIR recipients to the need to wash all cans and reduce the risk of leptospirosis.

Write the full text of the anti-leptospirosis message that you would include in the bag of canned foods. Needs assessment data indicate that Native Americans have a high school dropout rate of 50%, compared to 30% for the non-Native population. Be sure that your message is designed for those who have not graduated from high school. To increase the likelihood of adoption of the recommended behavior, offer a rationale for your message.

The message:

<u>Monitoring consumption of dried fruit intake</u>

For persons with diabetes and overweight and obese persons, one of the disadvantages of dried fruit is that overconsumption may lead to excessive sugar and _____ intake. It is easier to overconsume sugar and calories in smaller portions of dried fruit than in fresh fruit. A prune is a dried plum. A person is likely to eat _____ plum at one sitting. However, ½ cup of cooked prunes—more than 4 dried plums, is common. Few persons eat 4 _____ plums at one sitting.

	Sugar (teaspoons)	Calories
½ cup prunes, cooked	6	133
1 plum	1	30

Half a cup of cooked prunes has _____ times more sugar and _____ times more calories than a plum.

Tips on mindful eating would be relevant for FDPIR program participants, especially those who are overweight and obese and those who have been diagnosed with _____.

Chapter 7
Culturally Sensitive Needs Assessment

Planning a Sports Nutrition Program for the local high school Football Team
List 5 football terms and phrases:
1.
2.
3.
4.
5.

Using these football terms, develop a title which is related to their nutritional mistakes. Alliteration (Fibra Forever!), and questions, ("Are You on Your Way to 5 Fruits and Vegetables Today?") make for titivating titles.
1.
2.
3.

You are planning a 6-session Sports Nutrition program for the local high school football team.

Your needs assessment data (24-hour food recalls from five players) revealed that like most athletes, their nutritional mistakes include: underhydration, excessive fat intake, and inadequate carbohydrate intake. One parent of a football player who is an amateur sports nutritionist theorizes that whenever the game goes into overtime, the team loses--they run out of muscle glycogen due to inadequate carbohydrate intake.

For each of the following topics, identify one visual that you would use:

Sports Nutrition Topic	Visual that you would use with football players
Underhydration	
Excessive fat intake	
Inadequate CHO intake	

You are planning to conduct an 8-session nutrition program to increase fruit and vegetable intake among Mexican farm workers at their clinic. You call the largest clinic which serves Mexican farm workers. Write the text of your email for the nurse and the telephone message. Leave a blank line in between each line to accommodate revisions.

Text:

Telephone message:

Chapter 8
Culturally Sensitive Dietary Assessment

<u>Conduct a 24-hour food recall with a culturally different client</u>

Find a partner, and the taller person will be the interviewing RDN, and the shorter person will be the culturally different client.

*Instructions for Completing a 24-Hour Food Recall—**Taller Student***

*The taller student needs to review the following instructions to guide the shorter person to describe all the foods and beverages, and portion sizes that they had yesterday. Your purpose is to guide the client to help you to make a **complete** list of all foods and beverages for a typical day.*

1. *Include methods of preparation – raw, broiled, fried, baked*

   Form of food -   *buttered toast, whole milk, yogurt with fruit, meat trimmed of fat, cake with frosting*

   Condiments -   *ketchup, mustard, mayonnaise, salad dressing, cream or sugar in coffee, syrup on pancakes*

2. *Estimate the **PORTION** size:*

   By volume -   *Cups, tablespoons*

   By weight -   *Ounces, pounds*

   By unit -   *1 biscuit*

                       1 frankfurter

                       1 medium apple

3. *Ask about breakfast, lunch, dinner and snacks.*

4. *Explore ethnic food consumption—*
   "How is it usually prepared?
   "What do you usually add at the table?
   "What are some of your favorite ethnic foods…
   for Breakfast?
   for Lunch?
   for Dinner?
   for Snacks?
   for Dessert?

5. *"How often do you get to have your ethnic foods?*
   In response to an unfamiliar food:
   --"How do I spell that?"
   --"What does it taste like?"
   --"Where can I buy it?"
   --"How was it prepared?"

At some point during the interview, be sure to offer a deliberate inappropriate verbal or non-verbal response (What?, raised eyebrows or a frown) when the client mentions an unfamiliar ethnic food.

*Instructions for Reporting on Food and Beverage Intake--**Shorter Student***

For the purposes of this exercise, you are Mr. James or Mrs. Jan Santos, a Filipino American who eats mostly Filipino food. You do not cook. You often eat in Filipino restaurants.

When the registered dietitian nutritionist asks you to describe what you ate, you list the following Filipino foods and beverages. You describe meals and the **type of meat and "vegetables"**. You do not know foods are prepared. You drink jasmine and oolong tea. IF you are asked if it is sweetened, you reply "**with 2 teaspoons of sugar**".

Breakfast

-jasmine and oolong tea. "with 2 teaspoons of sugar"—ONLY if you are asked.

Lunch

-5 lumpia—4 or 5 spring rolls

-chicken adobado—1 chicken leg and thigh, vegetables

-rice, 2 cups

- jasmine and oolong tea. "with 2 teaspoons of sugar"—ONLY if you are asked.

Dinner

-siopao—3 steamed buns

-1 balut –Respond if asked with "fertilized duck egg"

-beef pancit—3 cups beef and noodles, vegetables ½ cup

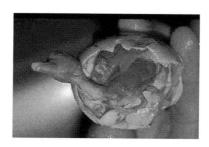 Filipino balut

After-Action Review Questions for RDN and client:

Clients:

1. Which negative non-verbal cues did you observe?

2. Which negative verbal comments did you observe?

3. Would you return for a follow-up consultation?

RDN:

1. What was the hardest part of the 24-hour recall?

2. What was the easiest part?

During a 24-hour recall, which column lists appropriate and inappropriate questions?

Column A
-What do you usually add at the table?
-What are some of your favorite ethnic foods for
Breakfast..., for Lunch..., for Dinner..., for Snacks?
-How was it prepared?
-Tell me more about that?

Column B
-Why did you eat that?
-What's that?
-What?
-Why did you prepare the
rice like that?

The Art of Apologizing

The purpose of the apology is to admit the mistake, soothe the client's jangled nerves, and to help the client to return to the goal of using mainstream and ethnic foods to solve the nutrition problem.

An apology should include the following components:
"I am so sorry about how I responded to your statement. I was surprised by your ethnic food.
-I didn't mean to show my surprise in that negative way. I don't know what I was thinking. Please forgive me. It won't happen again.
-It's important for me to find out about all the ethnic foods that you eat and drink so that I can guide you on which ones can be used to reverse your high blood pressure.
-The more I think about, the more I realize that all over the world people derive nutrients from foods that are different to American foods. I'll have to work on my cross-cultural IQ.
-Please, tell me more about the ethnic foods that you usually have for breakfast…lunch…dinner…snacks…desserts—even the unfamiliar ones!

RDN: In your own words, write the text of your apology for your negative non-verbal cue.

Identifying and responding to ethnic holidays

Culturally sensitive nutritionists make sure to consider ethnic holidays into nutrition programming two ways. First, to improve attendance at nutrition sessions, it is important to schedule nutrition programs **before or after** ethnic holidays. Scheduling a nutrition session during a holiday is likely to lead to _____ attendance. Planning nutrition programs WITH the target population is a sure way to schedule nutrition programs around them.

Second, providing nutrition education on healthy holiday eating prior to the holidays allows clients to make decisions _____ temptation strikes. For many adults and children who are at risk of overweight, overweight, or obese, ethnic holidays make it more difficult than usual to eat healthfully. Celebrating ethnic holidays with family members and loved ones, anticipating and overindulging in long-awaited high-fat, high-sugar holiday favorites are linked to weight gain, and poor glycemic control in persons with _____. Nutritionists who offer multiple healthy holiday eating tips make it easy for clients to _____ which tips would work for them. Preparing for healthful holiday eating is particularly valuable for overweight and obese clients, persons with diabetes, and for Muslims with diabetes who fast during daylight hours, and eat a meal after sunset during the _____ days of Ramadan.

At https://aes.wfu.edu/calendar-of-ethnic-holidays/,
1. Identify one unfamiliar ethnic holiday in your birth month.
2. From an Internet search, list two red light ethnic holiday foods.
3. For each food, offer two strategies to reduce the harmful effects of the holiday food.

Resources for Healthy Holiday Eating

-https://www.diabeteseducator.org/living-with-diabetes/spanish-resources

-https://www.heart.org/en/healthy-living/healthy-eating/eat-smart/nutrition-basics/holiday-healthy-eating-guide

Ethnic Holiday:
Red light ethnic holiday food 1: _____
1.
2.

Red light ethnic holiday food 2: _____
1.
2.

Chapter 9
Culturally Sensitive Nutrient Analysis

The purpose of culturally sensitive nutrient analysis is a) to determine the nutrient content of an ethnic foods, and b) to classify them as a red/yellow/green light food. In this way, clients can be guided to use the ethnic food, whether it is a red, yellow, or a green light food, to solve nutrition problems. Ethnic foods may be consumed as single foods—a fresh mango, or as combination foods which consist of multiple ingredients.

Helping Chinese American pregnant women to enjoy confinement soups

In many Asian countries, postpartum women are confined for 40 days. Chinese American women enjoy 'mothers' soup' immediately after childbirth. They are believed to cure too much cold (yin), shrink the womb, and decrease stagnant Chi (life force). There are more than 20 different types of Chinese confinement soups.

Case Study—Mrs. Shangyu Zhou

Mrs. Zhou usually has about 2 8-ounce cups of Pig's Feet with Ginger in Black Vinegar soup a day. She believes that the soup "removes 'wind' from the body, helps warm the body, provides iron and calcium from pigs' feet. As the pigs' feet boils, the marrow comes out of the bones into the soup. The black vinegar helps purify the blood and clears the arteries of stale blood".

Pig's Feet with Ginger in Black Vinegar

1 whole pig's feet, halved, cut into edible sections

10 large pieces of fresh ginger (5000 grams)

2 large bottles of sweet vinegar (1000 mL)

(Sweet balsamic vinegar of Modena)

1 large bottle of black rice vinegar (500 mL)

2 hard-boiled eggs

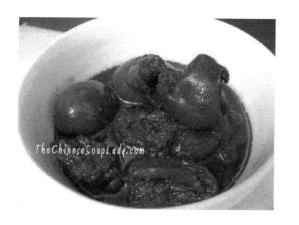

http://www.thechinesesouplady.com/pigs-feet-with-ginger-in-black-vinegar/

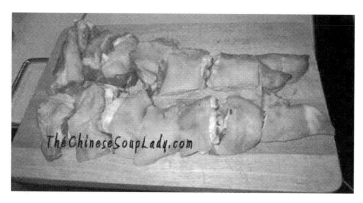

Analysis of Chinese mothers' soup:

To find the nutrient content of foods from

the USDA database, use the descriptor

USDA nutrient content pickled pigs' feet

Use the Nutrient Analysis Table to analyze the nutrient content of an ethnic combination food—1 cup of Chinese pig's feet with ginger in black vinegar:

Nutrient Analysis Table

For each ingredient: Nutrient content of each recipe ingredient; Reference portion sizes; Converted to the quantity in recipe; Source	Sugars (g)	Fats (g)	Saturated Fats (g)	Sodium (mg)
N R C S				

Nutrient Analysis Table--Pig's Feet with Ginger in Black Vinegar

Nutrient content of each recipe ingredient; reference portion sizes; converted to the quantity in recipe; source	Sugars (g)	Fats (g)	Saturated Fats (g)	Sodium (mg)
Nutrient content of **1 pigs' foot**? a. of reference portion size, 1 pigs' foot b. converted to the quantity in recipe https://www.fatsecret.com/calories-nutrition/generic/pork-pigs-feet-cooked	0 —	14 —	4 —	204 —
Nutrient content of **2 boiled eggs**? a. of reference portion size, 1 boiled egg b. converted to the quantity in recipe https://fdc.nal.usda.gov/fdc-app.html#/food-details/339005/nutrients	.2 —	4 —	1 —	189 —
Nutrient content of **sweet vinegar 1000 mL**? a. of reference portion size, 1 TBSP b. converted to quantity in recipe: How many TBSP in 1000mL? 1000mL=4.2 cups; 1 cup=16 TBSP; 4.2 cups=67 TBSP https://www.myfooddiary.com/foods/7324048/colavita-sweet-balsamic-vinegar-modena	3 —	0 —	0 —	0 —
Nutrient content of **black rice vinegar 500 mL**? a. of reference portion size, 100mL=2.1 cups b. converted to the quantity in recipe https://world.openfoodfacts.org/product/6902007508302/heng-shun-chinkiang-black-rice-vinegar	3 —	0 —	0 —	800 —
Total Nutrient Content in Recipe? Add "b" of all ingredients	—	—	—	—
Nutrient content in 1 cup= Total Volume/Portion Size Total volume (cups) of all ingredients? 1 pigs' foot, cooked, weighs 87g =.4 cup 2 boiled eggs weigh 88g =.4 cup Total volume of recipe=.4 cup pigs' foot + .4 cup boiled eggs + ginger + 4.2 cups sweet vinegar + 2.1 cups black rice vinegar=7.1 cups TOTAL NUTRIENT CONTENT in 1 cup/7.1	—	—	—	____mg= ____g

To determine if pigs' feet with ginger in black vinegar is a red/yellow/green light food, use the traffic light food classification table:

	Sugars (g)	Fat (g)	Saturated Fats (g)	Sodium (1g=1000mg)
1. Client's nutrient intake, **1 cup** (Use 2 decimal points for each nutrient)				
Red light foods	>15	>20	>5	>1.5
Yellow light foods	5-15	3-20	1.5-5	0.3-1.5
Green light foods	<5	<3	<1.5	<0.3
1 cup of _____ is classified as a _____ light food.				
2. Nutrient content in **.4 cup**=the Client's Portion Size Factor CPSF=.4/1=.4 * Line 1 (Use 2 decimal points for each nutrient)				
Red light foods	>15	>20	>5	>1.5
Yellow light foods	5-15	3-20	1.5-5	0.3-1.5
Green light foods	<5	<3	<1.5	<0.3

If the client had **.4 cup** of _____, it would be classified as a _____ light food.

The Traffic Light Food Classification table for Pig's Feet with Ginger in Black Vinegar

	Sugars (g)	Fat (g)	Saturated Fats (g)	Sodium (1g=1000mg)
1. Mrs. Zhou had **1 cup** (Use 2 decimal points for each nutrient)	30.42	3.10	.85	.75
Red light foods	>15	>20	>5	>1.5
Yellow light foods	5-15	3-20	1.5-5	0.3-1.5
Green light foods	<5	<3	<1.5	<0.3

1 cup of Pig's Feet with Ginger in Black Vinegar confinement soup is classified as a _____ light food.

	Sugars (g)	Fat (g)	Saturated Fats (g)	Sodium (1g=1000mg)
2. Nutrient content in **.4 cup**=the Client's Portion Size Factor CPSF=.4/1=.4 * Line 1 (Use 2 decimal points for each nutrient)	12.17	1.24	.34	.30
Red light foods	>15	>20	>5	>1.5
Yellow light foods	5-15	3-20	1.5-5	0.3-1.5
Green light foods	<5	<3	<1.5	<0.3

If Mrs. Zhou had **.4 cup** of Pig's Feet with Ginger in Black Vinegar confinement soup, it would be it would be classified as a _____ light food.

If Mrs. Zhou had 2 cups of soup, that would be classified as a _____ light food:

	Sugars (g)	Fat (g)	Saturated Fats (g)	Sodium (1g=1000mg)
1. Client's nutrient intake, **1 cup** (Use 2 decimal points for each nutrient)	30.42	3.10	.85	.75
2 cups	——	——	——	——
Red light foods	>15	>20	>5	>1.5
Yellow light foods	5-15	3-20	1.5-5	0.3-1.5
Green light foods	<5	<3	<1.5	<0.3

Mrs. Zhou usually has 2 8-ounce servings of this soup a day. Offer three recommendations that she could use to make mothers' soup more nutritious.

1.

2.

3.

Discovering that all empanadas are not made equal!
Empanadas--deep fried or baked flour dough with different fillings--are popular among Puerto Ricans, Venezuelans, and Colombians.

During a consultation, Senora Ruiz, an overweight Venezuelan client, states that she does not cook. She lives with her daughter who loves to cook. She states: "Then I had an empanada!"
An Internet search with the descriptor:
nutrient content types of empanadas
generates this table:

Type of Empanada	Calories	Fat (g)	CHO (g)	PRO (g)
Beef (Goya)	263	17	20	7
Chicken	235	14	21	8
Chicken Empanada (Red Ribbon)	261	17	22	7
Vegetable	193	11	20	5
Cheese	273	17	21	9
Fruit-Filled Mexican	452	25	55	4
Pumpkin Empanada (Taco Time)	256	8	42	6
Cherry Empanada (Mighty Taco)	190	6	31	3

Nutrient analysis often provides surprises when different types of food items are explored. The empanada with the highest fat content is the _____ empanada; and the lowest fat empanada is the _____ empanada.

A culturally sensitive nutritionist offers multiple strategies for reducing the harmful effects of the red light and yellow light ethnic foods, and for incorporating more green light ethnic foods to solve the client's nutrition problems. Prohibitions of ethnic and mainstream foods are unlikely to be successful in the short- or long-term, and may reduce the likelihood of follow-up _____. Clients have decades of conditioning, and fond _____ which are associated with ethnic foods, no matter how harmful they are. Even sharing the health risks of red light ethnic foods are not likely to lead to abandonment of red light ethnic foods. Instead of explaining "Empanadas because they have so much fat that they increase your blood _____ levels, and your risk of having a heart attack", offer recommendations:

1. for reducing portion size, frequency of ethnic red and yellow light foods
2. for liberal intake of ethnic and mainstream _____ light foods
3. for _____ intake of anti-inflammatory foods
4. eating green light and anti-inflammatory foods BEFORE eating red and _____ light foods.

Potential responses to Senora Ruiz:

1. What _____ of empanada do you usually have?

2. Which is the appropriate question that you would use for Senora Ruiz:

A. Where did you have the empanada?

or

B. How was your empanada prepared?

3. Presenting take-home list of anti-inflammatory foods…

  "Senora Ruiz, would you consider…

…eating more anti-inflammatory foods (green leafy vegetables, salmon, mackerel, herring, ground flaxseed)? They can help to minimize the effect of the cholesterol-r_____ saturated fat in the beef empanada.

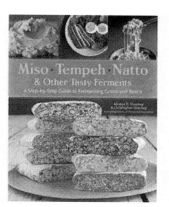

<u>Anti-inflammatory foods</u>
-**green** foods--mustard greens, turnip greens, collard greens, parsley, cilantro, arugula
-**purple** foods--Concord grapes and grape juice; red grapes, plums, prunes, eggplant, acai berries, blackberries, black raspberries, blueberries
-**high-alkalinity** foods—cauliflower, kale, celery, cucumber, broccoli, spinach, red bell pepper
-**omega-3-rich** foods--mackerel, herring, wild-caught salmon; chia seeds, ground flaxseed, tofu; Japanese natto, miso, tempeh (fermented soy products).

Would you consider…

…eating more green light foods?

Do you see yourself adding 2 tablespoons of frozen _____ _____ _____ to rice, pasta, and potatoes?

Or would you add 1 tablespoon of frozen green leafy vegetables to omelets.

My favorite green smoothie is recipe is: 1 cup frozen spinach, 1 cup of pineapple.

What is your favorite _____? You could add equal amounts of frozen spinach and your favorite fruit for a quick smoothie.

Would you consider…
…trying the 50% Rule for portion size and _____? That way you could eat the beef empanada half as often, or you could eat half the usual portion size.

I have a heart healthy empanada recipe here, would you like to get it for your _____?
Find a heart-healthy recipe online and place it here:

Present the recipe to Mrs. Ruiz describing its benefits and your experience with that recipe. You would say….

Chapter 11
Ethnic Food Guide Pictorial Representations

<u>Comparing FGPRs</u>
Review the article on Canvas:

Painter J, Rah J, Lee Y. Comparison of International Food Guide Pictorial Representations. *Journal of the American Dietetic Association.* 2002;102(4). 483-489.

Answer the following questions:

1. Which country does not include milk and dairy products as a food group?

2. Which is the only country which has a fluid group in its FGPR?

3. Identify one FGPR. If there was one feature that you would change, what would it be? Respond in 2 lines, 12 font. Include a visual to support your rationale.

Sample Response:

India: Since India has multiple regional cuisines, I recommend including a FGPR for each regional cuisine.

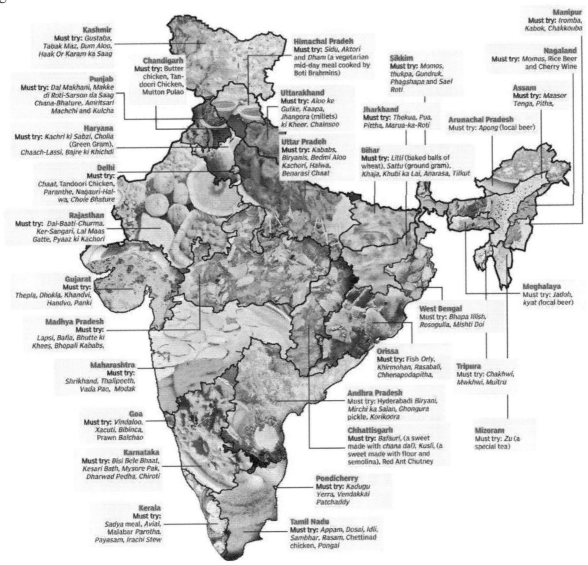

Manipur
Must try: *Iromba, Kabok, Chakkouba*

Kashmir
Must try: *Gustaba, Tabak Maz, Dum Aloo, Haak Or Karam ka Saag*

Himachal Pradesh
Must try: *Sidu, Aktori* and *Dham* (a vegetarian mid-day meal cooked by Boti Brahmins)

Sikkim
Must try: *Momos, thukpa, Gundruk, Phagshapa and Sael Roti*

Nagaland
Must try: *Momos*, Rice Beer and Cherry Wine

Chandigarh
Must try: Butter chicken, Tandoori Chicken, Mutton Pulao

Punjab
Must try: *Dal Makhani, Makke di Roti-Sarson da Saag Chana-Bhature, Amritsari Machchi and Kulcha*

Uttarakhand
Must try: *Aloo ke Gutke, Kaapa, Jhangora* (millets) *ki Kheer, Chainsoo*

Jharkhand
Must try: *Thekua, Pua, Pittha, Marua-ka-Roti*

Assam
Must try: *Maasor Tenga, Pitha,*

Haryana
Must try: *Kachri ki Sabzi, Cholia* (Green Gram), *Chaach-Lassi, Bajre ki Khichdi*

Uttar Pradesh
Must try: *Kababs, Biryanis, Bedmi Aloo Kachori, Halwa, Benarasi Chaat*

Bihar
Must try: *Litti* (baked balls of wheat), *Sattu* (ground gram), *Khaja, Khubi ka Lai, Anarasa, Tilkut*

Arunachal Pradesh
Must try: *Apong* (local beer)

Delhi
Must try: *Chaat*, Tandoori Chicken, Paranthe, Nagauri-Halwa, Chole Bhature

Rajasthan
Must try: *Dal-Baati-Churma, Ker-Sangari, Lal Maas Gatte, Pyaaz ki Kachori*

Meghalaya
Must try: *Jadoh, kyat* (local beer)

Gujarat
Must try: *Thepla, Dhokla, Khandvi, Handvo, Panki*

West Bengal
Must try: *Bhapa Illish, Rosogulla, Mishti Doi*

Madhya Pradesh
Must try: *Lapsi, Bafla, Bhutte ki Khees, Bhopali Kababs,*

Orissa
Must try: Fish *Orly, Khirmohan, Rasabali, Chhenapodapitha,*

Tripura
Must try: *Chakhwi, Mwkhwi, Muitru*

Maharashtra
Must try: *Shrikhand, Thalipeeth, Vada Pao, Modak*

Andhra Pradesh
Must try: Hyderabadi *Biryani, Mirchi ka Salan, Ghongura* pickle, *Korikoora*

Mizoram
Must try: *Zu* (a special tea)

Goa
Must try: *Vindaloo, Xacuti, Bibinca, Prawn Balchao*

Chhattisgarh
Must try: *Bafauri,* (a sweet made with *chana dal*), *Kusli,* (a sweet made with flour and semolina), Red Ant Chutney

Karnataka
Must try: *Bisi Bele Bhaat, Kesari Bath, Mysore Pak, Dharwad Pedha, Chiroti*

Pondicherry
Must try: *Kadugu Yerra, Vendakkai Patchaddy*

Kerala
Must try: *Sadya* meal, *Avial, Malabar Parotha, Payasam, Irachi Stew*

Tamil Nadu
Must try: *Appam, Dosai, Idli, Sambhar, Rasam,* Chettinad chicken, *Pongal*

Recommendations for improving the next edition of the Mexican FGPR

You have secured a consultancy with the Mexican government to review and make recommendations on the next edition of the Mexican FGPR. The last edition was in 2015. For many White and non-White persons, coping with holiday eating is a topic of perennial interest. Review three typical Mexican breakfasts, and Mexican Christmas foods below.

Review the Mexican FGPR at:

http://www.fao.org/nutrition/education/food-based-dietary-guidelines/regions/countries/mexico/en/

Make two specific recommendations to the Mexican Food Guide Pictorial Representation Committee for the next edition. Offer the rationale for each recommendation. Using the format below, the recommendation should not 3 lines.

I recommend *the inclusion of the most popular prepared dishes, and fewer single foods.* ***This would*** *allow users to relate their meals to the FGPR.*

Format:
"I recommend _____. This would _____."

1.

2.

Three Typical Mexican Breakfasts

- **Huevos Rancheros**: lightly fried corn tortilla and fried eggs with a sauce made from peppers, tomatoes, onions, garlic and pepper blended altogether (usually served with refried beans as well).

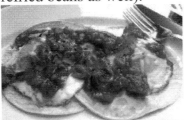

- **Chicharron con chile**: chicharrones (fried pork rinds) cooked with a sauce made from roasted tomatoes, roasted peppers, garlic and salt.

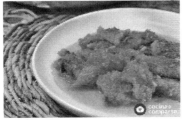

- **Sopitas con huevo**: fried corn tortillas cooked with eggs. Usually served with sour cream.

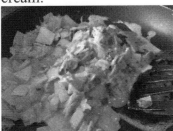

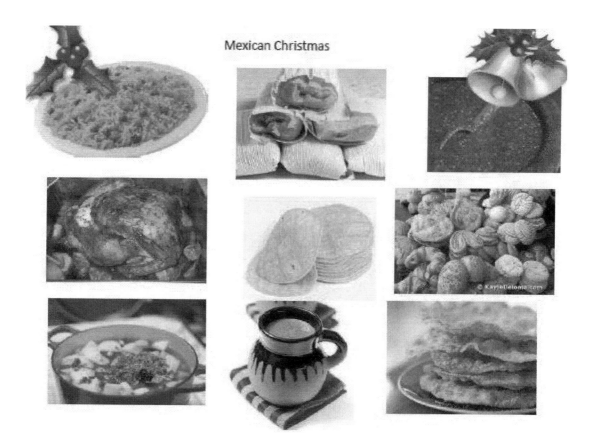

Mexican Christmas

Evaluating two Arab language FGPR

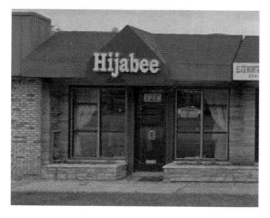

Dearborn, Michigan has the highest percentage of Muslim Americans in the country. Among those classified as Whites in Dearborn, Michigan, a suburb of Detroit, 41% of Whites are Arab Americans. Stores such as Hijabee, hookah cafes, Muslim women wearing hijabs and floor length dresses are tell-tale signs of the large Muslim population. Nationwide, the majority of Arab Americans have ancestral ties to Lebanon, Syria, Palestine, Egypt and Iraq (Arab American Institute, 2019).

1. Identify two potential Arab language FGPR.
2. Evaluate both FGPRs, and select the one that you would use during a 5-A-Day program with the Arab American Chamber of Commerce. State the rationale for your choice in less than 2 lines.

On one page, place both FGPRs.
Arab language FGPR 1:

Arab language FGPR 2:

I would use .... because it has the following two strengths:
A.
B.

Chapter 12
Culturally Sensitive Diet Counseling

Self-Awareness Activity

Enter the first three words that come to mind when you hear the following words:
Homeless people are:
1.
2.
3.

Hispanics are:
1.
2.
3.

Guiding Japanese Americans to use Japanese foods to reverse nutrition problems

In Japanese cuisine,

-shrimp, sweet potato, green pepper tempura are …………light foods;

-miso soup (miso is fermented soy paste) is a ……………… light food, and

-a raw salad of red cabbage, cherry tomato, iceberg lettuce, with ginger salad dressing is a

……….. light food.

To make tempura less inflammatory, you could

1.

2.

3.

To make high-sodium miso soup less inflammatory, you could:

1.

2.

3.

Selecting visuals for Dominican American pregnant women

Identify 5 visuals which would help Dominican American pregnant women to initiate

 breastfeeding within 30 minutes of birth.

1.

2.

3.

4.

5.

Preparing Dominican American women for Holiday Eating

It is November, and as a WIC nutritionist in a Dominican American neighborhood, you review the Dominican Christmas foods, and make three recommendations to respond to the pregnant womens' double whammy concern—pregnancy weight gain, and that holiday eating could lead to even more weight gain. Needs assessment data also indicate that among FL WIC mothers:

28.9 % were obese

25.7% were overweight

36.9% were normal weight (United States Department of Agriculture, 2019).

1.
2.
3.

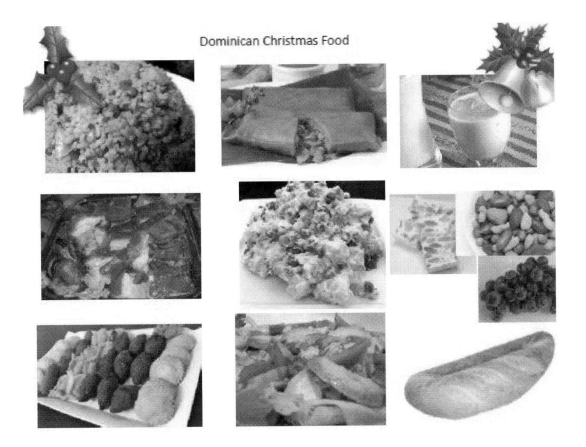

Dominican Christmas Food

Offer the Dominican Food Guide Pictorial Recommendation, describing one strength and one weakness:

"One of the strengths of the Dominican Food Guide Pictorial Recommendation is that:

-

One weakness is that:

-

Chapter 13
Culturally Sensitive Nutrition Lesson Planning

Weight Gain/Artery-Clogging/Pro-inflammatory
and
Weight loss/Heart-healthy/Anti-inflammatory dishes
from Multiple Cuisines

To ensure that clients leave a nutrition session with the discovery that
"I didn't realize that there were so many heart-healthy foods from other cuisines"
--culturally sensitive nutritionists share multiple weight loss/heart healthy/anti-inflammatory dishes from multiple cuisines.

For each of the following cuisines, identify the column listing weight gain/artery clogging/proinflammatory column, and the column listing weight loss/heart healthy/anti-inflammatory dishes.

Italian

Plain bread	Garlic Bread
Plain breadsticks	Fried Calamari
Salads with dressing on the side	Shrimp scampi
Lentil or minestrone soup	Cheese cannelloni, meat sauce
Baked clams	Spaghetti with meatballs
Fresh seafood	Fettuccine alfredo
	Chicken or eggplant parmigiana
Pasta with red clam, or wine sauce	Clam or white sauce
Pasta primavera	
Skim milk cappuccino	Pastries, cannoli, tiramisu

French

French bread	Croissant
Mussels	French onion soup
	En croute (wrapped in pastry)
Bouillabaisse (seafood stew)	Potatoes au gratin
Coq au vin (chicken stewed in wine)	Beef Bourguignon
Salad nicoise (dressing on the side)	Foie gras
Ratatouille	Quiche Lorraine
Pot au feu	Hollandaise,Bearnaise,Bechamelsauce
Quenelles (steamed fish dumplings))	Buerre blanc (butter sauce)
Mixed berries	Chocolate mousse
Sorbet	

Greek

Pita bread
Hummus, Olives
Chicken, fish
kabobs, souvlaki
Yogurt and cucumber salad
Greek salad without the dressing
Babaghanoush
Dolma (stuffed grape leaves)

Saganaki
Moussaka

Falafel in pita
Pastitsio
Gyro

Mexican

Soft flour tortillas
Sangria
Gazpacho
Bean soup
Bean chili
Bean, chicken, seafood fajitas or burritos
Salsa
Beans and rice
Taco salad without the shell

Tortilla chips, nachos
Margaritas

Refried beans
Chorizo (sausage)
Chimichanga (fried burrito)
Sour cream
Guacamole
Fried ice cream

Chinese

Clear soup

Hot-and-sour soup

Steamed vegetable, chicken, or shrimp dumplings

Steamed brown rice

Stir-fried or steamed chicken or seafood
  with vegetables

Chinese vegetables with tofu

Mu shu pork with no egg

Fortune cookies

Fried rice or noodles

Fried dumplings

Egg rolls, spring rolls

Spare ribs

Fried dishes

Sweet-and-sour dishes

Egg foo yung

Japanese

Edamame

Miso or su-udon soup

Sushi and sashimi

Mizutki (chicken, vegetables)

Tossed salad, miso dressing

Cucumber and seaweed salad

Steamed gyoza (shrimp dumplings)

Yosenabe (noodles, seafood, or vegetables
in broth); chicken, fish teriyaki

Tempura (fried food in batter)

Tonkatsu (fried pork cutlets)

Crispy fried noodles

Thai

Lime juice-based salads

Spring rolls in rice paper

Broth-based soups

Tom yum kunk (hot and sour soup)

Steamed dumplings

Chicken satay

Steamed white rice

Thai seafood salad

Thai chicken with basil

Green papaya salad

Mussaman beef curry

Thai coconut rice

Pad Thai

Thai beef salad

Thai coffee or tea

Indian

Chapati or puri bread

House Salad

Chicken tikka

Tandoori shrimp

Tandoori chicken without skin

Whole-wheat tandoori roti (without butter)

Bean and lentil stew (dal maharani)

Yogurt salad or raita

Green chutney

Roasted papadum (instead of fried)

Naan bread

Lamb korma (spicy curry)

Chicken curry

Vegetable fritters

Lamb biryani

Kulfi-faluda or gula jamun
(sweet, cream-filled dessert)

Vietnamese

Canh chua tom (spicy and sour shrimp soup)

Goi cuon (fresh spring roll)

Bo xa lui nuong (grilled beef with
lemon grass in rice paper with vegetables)

Ca hap (steamed whole fish)

Lychee (fruit in syrup)

Banh michien voitom (fried shrimp toast)

Vit quay (roast duck)

Cha gio (fried spring rolls)

Oy Heo xao chua ngot (sweet and sour pork)

Banh dua ca ra men (coconut flan with caramel)

Cajun (Louisana)

Boiled crawfish or shrimp

Creole and jambalaya dishes

Broiled or grilled seafood

Turkey or roast beef Po' Boy sandwiches

White rice

Red beans and rice without sausage

Fried crawfish or shrimp

Gumbo, etouffe and sauces made with roux

Fried seafood

Fried shrimp or oyster Po' Boy sandwiches

Dirty rice (chicken gizzards, livers, butter)

Red beans and rice with sausage

Activity--Local Ethnic Restaurants

List the names of 3 local Hispanic chain restaurants
1.
2.
3.

List the name of 3 local Caribbean chain restaurants
1.
2.
3.

List the name of 1 local Asian chain restaurant:
1.

Activity—Managing Program Eventualities--What Would You Do?

The Green Smoothie Competition was designed to help White and non-White university students increase fruit and vegetable intake. The president of the Student Dietetic Association arrived to host the Green Smoothie Competition with 120 pounds of fruits and vegetables and five blenders in the breezeway outside the library. But suddenly torrential rain began to fall, and the Organic Farmers' Market was cancelled. List 3 options for the Green Smoothie Competition under these circumstances.
1.
2.
3.

Despite the rain, the Green Smoothie Competition was held. It generated satisfied clients who were converted into Walking Talking billboards. They inquired:
"Are you a new organization?"
"Can we join if we're not in Nutrition?"
"Will you be here again?"
"This is better than Jamba Juice!"
"You guys should do this more often!"

FOOD SAFETY CASE STUDY

An Interactive 30-Minute Learning Experience

The Food Safety Case Study is presented after a 10-minute PowerPoint presentation which explained the five most common food safety mistakes, their consequences, and how to resolve them. In the Case Study, the client makes food safety mistakes and experiences the consequences. During the review of the case study, clients learn how to make sure that they do not make food safety mistakes or experience the same consequences.

Underline four food safety mistakes in the following case study.

For each mistake, describe the alternative appropriate food safety behavior.

Case Study

A few days before Thanksgiving, Carlos, who lives alone, decided to prepare his first Thanksgiving meal, invited a few friends over, and got ready to try his hand at cooking.

Carlos placed the 20# turkey on the kitchen counter to thaw it on Wednesday morning. The next day—Thursday, he cooked the turkey in the oven. He only had one cutting board so it was used for preparing all food items—stuffing, green beans, sweet potato casserole, and Caesar salad.

After 3 hours, Carlos took the steaming bird from the oven. When he started carving the turkey, it seemed a bit pink on the inside, but the aroma was wonderful. He had succeeded!

The meal was enjoyed by all, with everyone going back for seconds a few hours after the meal had been served.

Carlos was so proud of himself. However, the next day, all of Carlos' friends had to stay at home. They were having episodes of nausea, diarrhea, and vomiting! Carlos felt so guilty! He had no intention of hosting another Thanksgiving meal--ever.

Food Safety Case Study—Answer Key

Fill in the blanks in the table below.

This answer key can be shared with clients so that they can fill in the blanks in teams. The first team to complete the fill-in-the-blanks correctly wins a prize.

Hint (which would have been shared during the presentation): Allow at least 1 day of refrigerator thawing for every 4 pounds of turkey.

MISSTEPS	CONSEQUENCES	PREVENTION OF FOOD-BORNE ILLNESS
Carlos thawed the turkey on the counter	Bacteria divided rapidly at room temperature on the outer surface of the turkey	Thaw the turkey in the refrigerator, breast side up, in an unopened wrapper on a tray in the fridge. Therefore, Carols' 20-pound turkey needs ___ days to thaw in the fridge. Since Carlos planned to put the turkey in the oven on Thursday morning, he should have placed the turkey in the fridge to thaw on _____ (SSMTW).
He used one cutting board	Cross-contamination among four foods-- stuffing, green beans, sweet potato casserole, Caesar salad	Use a separate cutting board and utensils for _____ dish. Wash the cutting board after each food item. Use a cleanable acrylic, not wooden, cutting board.
Turkey was a bit pink inside and it was still served	Inadequately cooked turkey was contaminated with bacteria	Use a food thermometer to ensure that the turkey is cooked to a minimum internal temperature of 165 °F. Place the food thermometer at the innermost part of the thigh and wing, and at the _____ part of the breast.
Everyone went back for seconds a few hours after the meal	Higher bacterial content after a few hours.	Refrigerate all foods immediately to stop bacterial growth in all _____ contaminated foods-- turkey, sweet potato casserole, stuffing, and green beans

True/False Statements

Setting: Multiethnic Black men in barbershops.

Clients are given the True/False statements and are asked to choose True or False for each statement individually.

Then the nutrition educator reviews each statement, explaining the rationale for the True/False designation, and offering additional take-home information on where to get a free PSA test; recommended foods for reducing prostate cancer risk, the cheapest place to buy them, tasty ways to prepare them; and how to eat out and enjoy more of those foods.

Are You Powering Up your Prostate?

Put "T" if you think the statement is TRUE.

Put "F" if you think the statement is FALSE.

1._____ Black and White men die from prostate cancer at the same rates.

2._____ Black men have 13% more testosterone than White men.

3._____Cooked tomotoes, pink grapefruit, pink guava, and watermelon can improve the health of the prostate gland.

4._____The best way to reduce the chances of getting prostate cancer is to eat more fruits and veggies.

Take-Home Answer Key:

1. False. Black men are twice as likely to die from prostate cancer as White men. For every White man who dies, two Black men die.

2. True.

3.True. Cooked tomatoes have 20% more of a prostate-friendly pigment called lycopene than raw tomatoes.

4. False. The best way to reduce the chances of getting prostate cancer is to find out your risk of getting prostate cancer by doing a blood test which will tell you how much of a protein called prostate specific antigen, you have.

After sharing the correct responses with clients individually, ask clients if they would like to take the flyer with the correct responses home, for potential sharing with loved ones. In this way, loved ones are likely to be able to share the 'Ah-hah' moment which the client experienced when they got the response _____ during the nutrition education session. When loved ones review the flyer, this gives them the opportunity to become part of the plan for dietary improvement, and to become the client's _____.

Are You Bolstering Your Breast with Breast-Friendly Foods?
Supermarket Digital Scavenger Hunt

Setting: Multiethnic Hispanic church women

During a 10-minute PowerPoint presentation, Hispanic church women discover the anti-breast cancer foods, taste testing, and the c................... place to buy them. Then they will be ready for the Supermarket Digital Scavenger Hunt.

Instructions:
Create a team which has a maximum of three members.
The first team which returns with photos of all foods wins a prize. Do not bring the actual foods. We only need photos of the foods.

Supermarket Digital Scavenger Hunt—
Are You Bolstering Your Breast with Breast-Friendly Foods?

Instructions:
Identify a partner. The first team which brings a photo of each of the following anti-breast cancer foods is the winner.
Your prize: a $25 supermarket gift card for each partner.

- Turmeric (Indian recipes)
- Acai berries (Brazilian recipes)
- Ginger
- Garlic
- Broccoli (Chinese recipes)
- Cauliflower, Brussel Sprouts, or Bok Choy
- Cilantro, Parsley, Endive or Arugula
- Eggplant
- Plums
- Blueberries
- Salmon
- Natto
- Miso
- Tempeh
- Concord Grapes
- Ground Flaxseed (whole flaxseed is 20% less effective at reducing blood cholesterol)
- Cherries

Apart from Whole Foods Market, which other health food stores could host this activity?
a. any supermarket which sells half of these foods
b. any supermarket which sells all of these foods
c. the closest supermarket to the church

Which of the following population groups would not find this activity to be fun?
a. older adults at the local senior center
b. any group of women who have cell phones that can take photos
c. breast cancer support group

When would be a good time to schedule a Supermarket Digital Scavenger Hunt?
a. Saturdays, Sundays
b. lunch and dinner time on any day of the week
c. 10 am any weekday

Which documents should the learners take home from the digital scavenger hunt?
a. a list of breast-friendly foods
b. the store's weekly flyer
c. samples, and coupons of breast-friendly foods
d. the memory of the taste of deli seaweed salad
e. all of the above

Increasing Satiety (the feeling of fullness) with Minimum Calories

American adults and children, whether they are White or non-White, who have grown accustomed to the feeling of fullness from high fat meals at every meal often complain that a low-fat diet leaves them feel hungry. This is in stark contrast to the Japanese who believe that a person should eat until they are 80% full. Clients who complain that a low-fat diet is too difficult may benefit from guidelines on how to feel full with minimum calories.

For each of the following recommendations, select the more appropriate word which is separated by a "/":

1. Drink 1 cup of water at the beginning/end of the meal

2. Have a vegetable salad with non-fat or low-fat salad mayo/dressing

3. Have a clear soup like wonton at the beginning/end of the meal

4. Drink ½ teaspoon of baking soda, 8 ounces water but only if you have low/high blood pressure

5. Drink 1 teaspoon of apple cider vinegar (ACV) and 8 ounces water. ACV tablets are concentrated acetic acid. They are not recommended because they can promote/block stomach ulcers.

6. Take valerian root supplements

7. Take aloe tablets or drink unsweetened aloe drink which is available in oriental grocery stores.

8. Do any yoga neck poses especially the shoulder/foot stand. This massages the thyroid gland and depresses appetite.

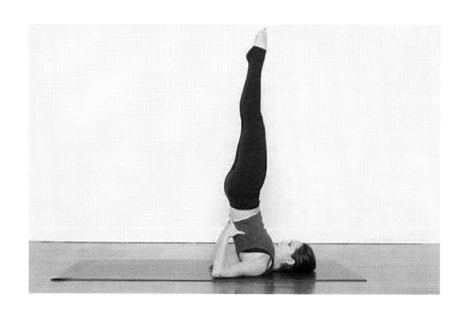

<u>Observing Eating Behavior</u>

Part 1

After you have finished a meal, go to a restaurant to observe peoples' eating behavior. If you are not hungry, it will be easier for you to observe others.

For 5 minutes, notice the extent to which restaurant patrons are:

1. eating and drinking at the same time. Do they put a beverage in the mouth although food is already in the mouth?

2. eating and adding more food. Do they add more food although food is already in the mouth?

3. eating quickly. How many times do they chew their food before swallowing?

4. eating and doing something else. Are they walking, watching TV, using their phones, or speaking while they are eating?

Based on your observation, what surprised you?

Part 2:

At your next meal, ask someone to observe you eating and answer the same 4 questions.

What could you do differently at your next meal?

What could you do so that it takes 20 minutes to finish eating a meal?

Personalizing Guidelines for Mindful Eating

<u>Sharing your experience of mindful eating</u>
To advocate mindful eating, it is important for the culturally sensitive nutritionist to have personal ………………in mindful eating.

<u>How Not to Advocate Mindful Eating</u>
When a client asks a nutritionist: *What's the worst part of mindful eating?*
The nutritionist replies *"You know, I'm not sure. I haven't tried it!"*

Clients are likely to remember a nutritionist's success story about overcoming obstacles to mindful eating. To recommend mindful eating means that the nutritionists needs to be, at least along the path to becoming a mindful _____. To build rapport with culturally different clients, recommend the guidelines, benefits of mindful eating, and share a personal ……………… about mindful eating. To be authentic, describe how you overcame _____ to mindful eating.

<u>Mastering mindful eating</u>

How long does it take for ………to finish a meal? Time yourself to see how long it takes you to finish your ……… meal. Ideally, it should take _____ minutes to finish a meal. Whether you have eaten 300 or 3000 calories, after 20 minutes, the stomach sends a message to the brain to say that the stomach is …………. An easy way to increase your eating time, is to use a timer to increase the time by 10%.

Eating mindfully—consciously focusing and enjoying food--can help you to reduce portion …………., enjoy more of each morsel, and condition you to develop a healthier relationship with food. The purpose is food is more to make your body healthier, than to make you _____ good.

Read the following guidelines of mindful eating and identify the easiest and the hardest ones for you.

1. The hardest mindful eating guideline for me to try would be:

2. The easiest mindful eating guideline for me to try would be:

List two environmental cues that you could use to increase your eating time, and to eat exclusively--without any other activity.

1.

2.

Guidelines for Mindful Eating

1. Sit down and unplug.

How to do it: Avoid watching TV and talking on the phone or texting while you eat. Stop working and step away from the computer. Set everything aside. Take a break to enjoy and savor your food. Focus on your meal.

How you'll benefit: Sitting down while you eat without distractions–will encourage you to pay attention to your food and how you consume it. You might find that you've fallen into a bad habit of eating too quickly or that you've been eating without tasting your food. And because mindful eating encourages you to take a true break, it can help you feel more relaxed or focused as you carry on with the rest of your day.

2. Eat slowly.

It takes the brain about 20 minutes to know that you've had enough food. Pausing in between bites can facilitate a healthy habit of eating slowly. Many people notice that if they have a sip of water in between each bite, that helps them to taste each morsel more fully.

How to do it: Set your fork down in between bites, for starters. Pause. Finish what's in your mouth before going for the next bite. Engage in stimulating conversation if you're eating with friends or family. Don't aim to get full. Be satisfied.

How you'll benefit: It's very likely that you'll eat a lot less. In this way, eating slowly helps prevent overeating, which causes unnecessary weight gain and digestive stress.

3. Chew well.

Eating on the run and devouring food without chewing very well can result in undigested food particles floating through the gut, bloating, gas and indigestion.

How to do it: Chew your food thoroughly until it has a fine, pulplike texture. Some experts suggest chewing each bite 30 to 50 times. Saliva is full of active enzymes that help break down food. The longer food is exposed to saliva (through chewing), the easier it moves through your intestines.

How you'll benefit: Proper chewing kickstarts the digestive process and allows for better absorption of vitamins and nutrients. Good digestion is essential for overall health.

4. Sip, don't gulp.

Drinking lots of water during meals can dilute your stomach acid, slowing down efficient digestion.

How to do it: Limit your consumption of fluids 15 minutes before you eat and for at least 15 to 30 minutes after a meal. If you prefer to drink with a meal, take small sips. Mint tea and lemon water are useful in assisting digestion.

How you'll benefit: By not flooding your system with excessive liquid, you can avoid or reduce gas and bloating. And you're likely to feel lighter after meals.

5. Embrace your senses.

Observe the colors, textures, aromas, sounds and the taste of each food is the best way to be fully present while eating.

How to do it: At your next meal, notice the colors and shapes of your food. Next, close your eyes and smell the aroma of your food. Keeping your eyes closed, what do noises do you hear? As you take a bite of food, notice the flavors and textures as you chew.

How you'll benefit: If you take the time to acknowledge and relish the colors flavors and textures of your food, you might be surprised at how certain sensory experiences begin to stand out. Embracing your senses at meals will also encourage you to slow down and enjoy the full experience of eating.

6. Eat only when you're hungry.

Eating when you're not hungry can lead to feeling guilty later about overeating. If you're hungry, of course, a healthy snack in between meals can be enjoyable and nourishing.

How to do it: Listen to your body. Is your stomach growling? Do you feel empty or light-headed? Are you thirsty? If you're truly hungry, eat a meal or have a healthy snack. Don't wait until you're famished and don't eat just because there is food around. When you grab a snack, ask yourself why you want it before you consume it.

How you'll benefit: Eating only when you're hungry serves as a reminder that your body needs energy and that you should for good health. Avoiding emotional eating and mindless snacking will keep those guilty feelings away as you move into mealtime. Eating only when you're hungry may help you avoid excessive weight gain.

7. Adopt an attitude of gratitude.

Acknowledge the time and effort put into creating your meal. Take a moment to consider all the hands that planted the food and how it moved the foods from farm to table.

How to do it: Take a moment to appreciate the nourishing, enjoyable aspects of your meal that you're about to indulge in. Say a blessing or simply pause to acknowledge your good fortune before the meal. Thank the person who prepared the food.

How you'll benefit: Everyone appreciates being acknowledged for their work and effort, and expressing gratitude at meals reminds us how people and nature connect to sustain us with nourishing food. This simple acknowledgement helps promote mindful eating habits and feelings of satisfaction all around.

Eating mindfully is a natural and pleasurable experience that supports good health. Your whole body will benefit from slowing down and being present while eating. It's not just what you eat, but *how* you eat that matters.

Adapted from: http://www.onemedical.com
One Medical Group, an innovative primary care practice with offices in Boston, Chicago, Los Angeles, New York, Phoenix, the San Francisco Bay Area, and Washington, DC.

Experiencing Mindful Eating

To experience mindful eating, bring a raisin to participate in the exercise in the Mindful Eating video at:

https://www.youtube.com/watch?v=C_IrfyjP88w

What surprised you about the experience?

Advocating Anti-Inflammatory Foods

Anti-inflammatory foods are some of the most beneficial foods because they reduce inflammation throughout the body in the arteries, gums, and bladder. Clients are more receptive to food recommendations than food prohibitions.

A........................ Anthocyanidin-Rich Foods

Food	Anthocyanidin content (mg/100 gram) 100 gram= 1/3 cup
Purple corn	1642
Elderberries	485
Acai	320
Purple carrots	169
Blueberries	163
Purple potatoes	159
Blackberries	100
Eggplant with skin	86
Blue corn	65-105
Red grapes	46
Red onions	10
Plums	6
Figs	0.5

There is no RDA for anthocyanidin.

Non-Purple .... Foods

*Fruits and vegetables which are deep green; and apples, pears, grapefruit; alfalfa
*1/2 a fresh pineapple/day
*Vegetables: spinach, kale, broccoli sprouts, cabbage, Bok choy/Pak choy, cauliflower
*Mushrooms—shiitake, reishi

*Fermented soy—natto, miso, tempeh, soy sauces; fermented tofu
*Nuts (65% fat): almonds, walnuts, hazelnuts; sunflower and pumpkin seeds

*Ginger (blended and strained three times, or cooked with meals)
*Spices: turmeric, fenugreek, cloves, allspice, nutmeg, bay leaf, cayenne, chili powder, red pepper flakes
*Garlic (Before eating, cut and leave exposed for 5 minutes to maximize effectiveness)
*Any peas and beans: chickpeas/garbanzo beans, kidney, pinto, navy, black beans; lentils, mung beans.

Foods that are rich in ....

Animal sources--salmon, herring, mackerel, sardines, sablefish, anchovies, cod liver oil

Plant sources--ground flaxseed, raw nuts and seeds, legumes
    Oils: almond, walnut, flaxseed
    Oils: borage, grapeseed, primrose, sesame, soybean

Flaxseed oil is particularly sensitive to heat, it needs to be refrigerated. To safeguard its flavor, it should not be heated before and during food preparation.

Your two favorite recipes for flaxseed oil are:

a.

b.

Chapter 14
Planning Culturally Sensitive Nutrition Programs

<u>Monthly National Health-Related Observances</u>

In a group of two students,

A. review the monthly national health-related observances and identify the nutrition-related observances for the birth month of each student at:
https://healthfinder.gov/nho/nhoyear.aspx?year=2018.
A. nutrition-related observance is any condition or ethnic group which you could target for nutrition programming. In the nutrition program, clients will be guided to use foods to reduce their risk of the condition.

B. choose one nutrition-related observance and ethnic group which has a higher prevalence of a nutrition-related condition.

C. create a title for one nutrition program for that ethnic group.

D. identify an already existing ethnic group which could be targeted for nutrition services.

E. References (AMA style).

FORMAT	SAMPLE
A. _____(month) is _____ (national nutrition-related observance month).	A. January is National Birth Defects Prevention Month.
B. Since _____ had a higher prevalence of _____ than Whites (Author, year),	B. Since American Indians/Alaska Natives had a 50% or greater prevalence for seven common birth defects (cleft lip, trisomy 18, and encephalocele, and lower, upper, and any limb deficiency) than non-American Indians/Alaska Natives (Canfield, Mai, Wang et al., 2014),
C. we would develop a nutrition proposal— _____ (title of nutrition program) for the:	C. we would develop a nutrition proposal— "Conquering Birth Defects—the Seminole Way!" (The Seminole Tribe of Florida call themselves "The Unconquered Tribe," because they never signed a peace treaty with the United States government. Between 1817 and 1858, the Seminoles fought three wars with U.S. troops.)
D. for the _____ (name, address of ethnic group).	D. for the: First Seminole Baptist Church, 4701 Stirling Rd, Hollywood FL
E. Reference (AMA style)	E. Canfield MA, Mai CT, Wang Y, O'Halloran M, Marengo LK, Olney RS, Borger CL, Rutkowski R, Fornoff J, Irwin N, Copeland G, Flood TJ, Meyer RE, Rickard R, Alverson CJ, Sweatlock J, Kirby RS. The Association Between Race/Ethnicity and Major Birth Defects in the United States, 1999-2007. American Journal of Public Health. 2014 104(9):e14-23. doi: 10.2105/AJPH.2014.302098. Accessed November 28, 2019.

Planners of a nutrition program should assume that clients are more like those described in columns A or B?

A	B
White clients are...	**White clients are...**
Excited to hear that some foods can reverse nutrition problems	Unaware of anyone who has ever reversed a nutrition condition
Thrilled about the options of buying new foods	Convinced that disease is due to fate and that you have to live with your disease
Anxious to try new foods	Overestimating diet quality
Willing to buy the recommended foods in a health food store	Overestimating nutrition knowledge
Aware of their barriers to dietary change, and are willing to try strategies to overcome them	Content to take their medication so that they can continue to eat their favorite foods
Are anxious to try new foods	Unaware of their barriers to dietary change—time, cost, convenience, habit, temptation—and unaware of strategies to overcome these barriers
	Not interested in changing any eating behaviors
Non-White clients...	**Non-White clients...**
Welcome the idea of abandoning their ethnic foods and eating more mainstream healthy foods—fruits and vegetables, low-fat dairy, peas and beans	Want to know how their red, yellow, and green light ethnic foods can be used to solve nutrition problems
Eat only ethnic foods	Eat a combination of traditional and ethnic foods

Activity—Hispanic Nutrition Program Planning

What Would Not Work? For each of the following Hispanic health and cultural norms, identify the inappropriate program feature in a 6-session church weight loss program?

IF THE HISPANIC CULTURAL NORM IS...	...THEN AN INAPPROPRIATE PROGRAM FEATURE WOULD BE...
1.Church members are from Central America, the Hispanic Caribbean, South American countries.	a. Place a different Hispanic flag on each PPT slide. b. Showcase ethnic superfoods from multiple Hispanic ethnicities. c. Host a session: Eating Right.
2. Curanderos (physical, mental, spiritual healers), espiritualistas (female faith healers), parteras (lay midwives), senoras (lay peer health educators) are traditional healers.	a. Ask traditional healers to advertise the nutrition program. b. Ask female healers to speak at the nutrition program. c. Send an email blast advertising the nutrition program to botanica customers.
3.Botanicas sell candles, statues, teas, prayers, amulets for healing rituals.	a. Invite botanica staff to speak at the nutrition program. b. Ask botanica staff to advertise the nutrition program. c. Request the botanica's mailing and email list.
4.Cuban American poverty rate is eight times lower than the Mexican American poverty rate. As household income increases, obesity rates decrease.	a. Target Mexican American churches for nutrition education. b. Target Cuban American churches for nutrition education. c. Recommend WIC and SNAP/Food Stamps programs to Mexican American congregations.
5.Horchata (sugar, milk, strawberry syrup), flan, tres leches, churros, chicharrones are favorite foods.	a. Share prohibitions on red light Mexican foods. b. Recommend the 50% Rule for red light Mexican foods, and share guidelines for mindful eating. c. Recommend eating 5 servings of fruits and vegetables before eating red light foods.
6.One family member's health problem calls for solutions from other family members.	a. Offer nutrition activities for seniors, adults, teens, children. b. Share a list of prohibited foods with obese family members. c. To cut back on calories, recommend drinking water at the beginning of meals.
7.Fatalism--disease is destiny, it is caused by misdeeds, or is pre-ordained, and individuals cannot influence the course of disease.	a. Share visual testimonials with pre-post health data, and describe how they overcame dietary obstacles. b. Offer multiple strategies for overcoming dietary obstacles. c. Recommend that clients go to Confession more often.
8.Beans are superfoods	a. Recommend beans for breakfast, lunch, dinner, snacks. b. Recommend rinsing canned beans. c. Recommend adding salt to canned beans to increase their shelf life.

Activity--Nutrition Program Planning with Hispanic Americans

Your nutrition consulting group has secured a consultancy with El Nuevo Heraldo (the Spanish edition of The Miami Herald) to launch a county-wide 5-A-Day campaign during Hispanic Heritage Month 15 Sep to 15 Oct. These days, newspaper sales are down because more consumers are getting their news on the Internet, and the Herald is anxious to increase subscriptions.

List 10 potential co-sponsors of the planning committee:

-

-

-

-

-

To the following list of 30-minute interactive learning experiences, add 2 additional team nutrition learning experiences by identifying traditional Hispanic recreational activities, and adapt them to nutrition team learning experiences. A team activity is likely to engage all learners. State the name of the Hispanic country and describe how the learning experience would work in 3 lines, with this format:

Country—to play....

Mexico—To play nutrition balero (a ball and cup game), when each team member answers a nutrition question correctly, that team member attempts to get the ball in the cup. The winning team gets the ball in the cup in the smaller number of attempts.

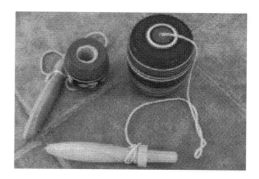

Supermarket tour
Ethnic grocery tour
Nutrition dominoes
Virtual restaurant tour
Nutrition Bingo
Nutrition Scattegories
Nutrition Jeopardy
Recipe Contest
True/False questions
Nutrition Scavenger Hunt
Food Label Comparison
1.
2.

Planning a Fiber Program at a Mexican American Senior Center

Needs assessment data indicate that some of their favorite Mexican foods are: nopales (cactus), jicama (starchy root tuber like potato), horchata (milk, sugar, chocolate, strawberry or other flavoring), tres leches (cake made with three types of milk--whole milk, condensed milk, evaporated milk), flan (sugar, egg yolks).

1. Which is the inappropriate RDN response:

a. "I'm not as familiar as I'd like to be with Mexican foods. Tell me more about horchata. What's it made from?"
b. "Oh, I really like Mexican food" (although you've never tried it)
c. "How often do you eat your ethnic foods?"
d. "How do you usually prepare nopales?"
e. "What is a typical portion size for you?"

2. Do you classify this Cactus Salsa recipe as a red/yellow/green light food?
2 cups nopales
2 cans diced tomatoes
 3 pickled jalapeno peppers
3 cloves
½ onion
1 15 oz. can red beans
1 15 oz, can black beans
1 15 oz. can pinto beans
A pinch of basil
¼ c olive oil
A dash of salt
A dash of black pepper
A tablespoon of sunflower seeds, shelled pumpkin seeds, pine nuts

3. Do you classify this French Fried Nopales recipe as a red/yellow/green light food?
1 pound fresh fava beans, shelled
1 pound fresh prickly pear cactus paddles/nopales
2 tablespoons olive oil
6 plum tomatoes, cut in half lengthwise
1 white onion, coarsely chopped
4 garlic cloves
2 red jalapeno chilies, thinly sliced
6 cups low-sodium chicken stock
1/4 cup coarsely chopped fresh cilantro

4. What type of milk would you recommend as an anti-inflammatory alternative to strawberry horchata--made with whole milk and strawberry syrup--for an overweight Mexican American client? Frozen strawberries with honey and
a. almond, rice, hemp, soy, or cashew milk
b. 2% milk
c. evaporated milk

5. How do you classify this Fava Bean and Nopales Soup recipe as a red/yellow/green light food?
1 pound fresh fava beans, shelled
1 pound fresh prickly pear cactus paddles/nopales
2 tablespoons olive oil
6 plum tomatoes, cut in half lengthwise
1 white onion, coarsely chopped
4 garlic cloves
2 red jalapeno chilies, thinly sliced
6 cups low-sodium chicken stock
1/4 cup coarsely chopped fresh cilantro

What Would Not Work? For each of the following multiethnic Black health and cultural norms, choose the inappropriate program feature in a 6-session church weight loss program?

Multiethnic Black Norms	Program Feature
1.Multiethnic Blacks include Haitian Americans, Caribbean Americans, African Americans, Africans from Africa.	Schedule a. Nutrition Dominos for Caribbean American men clients b. Nutrition Reggae Girlz Soccer team activity c. 1-hour nutrition lecture
2.Medical distrust of the Centers for Disease Control and Prevention (CDC) and their educational materials among African Americans because.	a. Share documents from CDC and explain: "I realize that the Centers for Disease Control and Prevention was responsible for the 70-year Tuskegee Experiment, and there has been a long history of medical malpractice with African Americans. However, I have reviewed this document and I think that it can help you to meet your dietary goals of eating more fruits and vegetables". b. Do not use CDC nutrition education materials with Blacks c. Explain that the CDC has changed and now all CDC educational materials like informed consent forms are written at 5th grade level.
3.Non-church gatherings begin with prayer	a. Before the meetings, find out who could say the prayer b. At the meetings, ask who would like to say the prayer c. No need to begin with prayer, it's a nutrition program
4.Blacks have lower health literacy levels than Whites	a. Use 5-A-Day brochures from the Internet. b. Adapt educational materials by using more white spaces, colors and visuals. c. Adapt materials so that they are written at the appropriate reading level.
5.HBCU Historically Black Colleges and Universities	Offer a session with the title: a. **H**ealthier? **B**ecause **C**alories **U**nderestimated =Trouble! b. On Your Way to 5 Fruits and Veggies a Day—the HBCU Way! c. More Sole Foods

Multiethnic Black Norms	Program Feature
6."The Divine Nine" is a group of African American fraternities and sororities; the Masons, Links; National Association for the Advancement of Colored People, National Urban League	a. Because women are food gate keepers, invite sororities, but not fraternities, to co-sponsor the weight loss program b. Invite male and female groups to co-sponsor the weight loss program c. Invite the all-male Masons to the weight loss program
7.History of family reunions	At the family reunion, schedule a. Learning activities for all age groups b. Activities with seniors exclusively because they have more health problems than others c. nutrition word searches and crossword puzzles
8.Less likely to drive a car than Whites	a. Arrange carpools to supermarket tour b. Coordinate church bus transportation to nutrition program c. Assume that transportation is not a problem because they make it to the movies okay
9.Grandma is the food gate keeper—she shops for food, cooks, and prides herself on her cooking.	Target: a. the Mothers' Union for nutrition education b. the Mens' Choir for nutrition education c. all church members for nutrition education
10.Fatback; pickled eggs, pigs' feet, sausage; fruit drinks, chitlins/chitterlings, hot fries are favorites.	a. Warn clients to stop eating these foods because of their excessive fat, sodium, or sugar content b. Recommend the 50% Rule in portion size with these foods c. Recommend the 50% Rule in frequency with these foods
11.Earn 30% less than Whites.	Schedule a session called: a.How to $tretch Your Food Dollar b.Why Coupons Aren't Worth the Trouble! c. Do You Qualify for WIC, SNAP, or congregate meal programs?
12.Collard greens are a top anti-cancer food	a.Promote collards for breakfast, lunch, dinner b.Recommend adding extra smoked meats to collards c.Recommend the cheapest places to buy collard greens

<u>Activity</u>--Nutrition Program Planning with Multiethnic Blacks

You have secured a consultancy with the local branch of the National Urban League Fort Lauderdale to conduct a 5-A-Day campaign during February--Black History Month.

List 10 potential co-sponsors of the planning committee:

-

-

-

-

-

To the following list of 30-minute interactive learning experiences, add 2 team nutrition learning experiences which are adapted from traditional recreational activities among African Americans, Caribbean Americans, Haitian Americans, and country-based Africans (Nigerian Americans).

Identify the country of interest, and traditional recreational activities. Adapt the recreational activity to a team nutrition learning experience.

State the name of the country and describe how the learning experience would work in 3 lines, with this format:

Country—to play….

Mexico—To play nutrition balero (a ball and cup game), when each team member answers a nutrition question correctly, that team member attempts to get the ball in the cup. The winning team gets the ball in the cup in the smaller number of attempts.

Supermarket tour
Ethnic grocery tour
Virtual restaurant tour
Nutrition Bingo
Nutrition Scattegories
Nutrition Jeopardy
Recipe Contest
True/False questions
Nutrition Scavenger Hunt
Food Label Comparison

African American nutrition learning experiences adapted from traditional recreational activities:

1.

2.

Caribbean American nutrition learning experiences adapted from traditional recreational activities:

1.

2.

Haitian American nutrition learning experiences adapted from traditional recreational activities:

1.

2.

Nigerian American nutrition learning experiences adapted from traditional recreational activities:

1.

2.

Nutrition Program Planning with Blacks

You are planning a 6-session nutrition program for Jamaican sugar cane farm workers in Belleglade, FL. For each of the following needs assessment data points, specify a program feature that you will include:

Needs Assessment Data	Program Feature
Median household income $22,715	
100% of sugar cane farm workers are Jamaican	

List…

A. 5 key informants for your XCNA
-
-
-
-
-

B. 3 1-hour nutrition activities which you would incorporate

-

-

-

C. 5 potential nutrition partners

-

-

-

-

-

D. List two strategies that could increase sales of the Jamaican restaurant owner who has become a co-sponsor:

-

-

E. List two evaluation questions that you would pose at the end of each session:

-

-

What Would Not Work? For each of the following multiethnic Asian health and cultural norms, choose the inappropriate program feature in a 6-session nutrition program?

Multiethnic Asian Norms	Program Feature
1.Southeast Asians are lactose intolerant.	Schedule a session called a. Top 10 Dairy-Free, High-Calcium Foods b. Eating Right c. How to Eat and Strengthen Your Bones
2.Laotians believe that 32 spirits oversee the body's 32 organs.	Schedule a session called a. The Top 32 Laotian Foods b. Eating Healthfully c. 32 Foods for 32 Organs
3.Among the Vietnamese, Cambodians, and Laotians, 60% of girls and 35% of boys have responsibility for preparing dinner	Target a. girls for nutrition education b. boys for leadership training, and girls for nutrition education c. boys for nutrition education
4.1 tablespoon of Vietnamese bone broth made with vinegar and bones offers as much calcium as 0.5 cup of milk	a. Prohibit the use of Dairy Ease and Lactaid (lactase supplements) b. Recommend liberal consumption of bone broth for breakfast, lunch, dinner, snacks c. Offer a session called "More Broth, Stronger Bones"
5.50-60% of Southeast Asian immigrants have tuberculosis (TB)have tuberculosis	a. Refer clients to Tai Chi practitioner for deep breathing techniques b. After a course of isoniazid (antibiotic that cures TB), recommend liberal consumption of anti-inflammatory green and purple foods for breakfast, lunch, dinner, snacks to reduce the risk of inflammation c. Remind clients to take isoniazid on an empty stomach for it to be effective.
6.The Hmong have the highest poverty rates and lowest English fluency among Southeast Asians	a. Offer low-literacy materials b. Emphasize Top 10 Most Nutritious Cheapest Foods c. Require English proficiency for nutrition education sessions
7.Strong family orientation to solving health problems	Target a. parents so that children learn kitchen skills in the teen years b. seniors because they are poly medicated and remind them of the importance of taking medication according to instructions c. seniors, adults, teens, children for different nutrition education activities

Multiethnic Asian Norms	Program Feature
8. Some Southeast Asian pregnant women are afraid that if they gain too much weight during pregnancy, the baby will grow too big, making delivery more painful.	a. Explain the Prenatal Weight Gain Grid and ask if she'd like to take it home and put it on her refrigerator door b. Do not allow mothers' Prenatal Weight Gain Grid to leave the clinic c. Describe the rationale for 25-pound weight gain (increase in breast size, blood volume, placenta…)
9. Every meal must contain rice. Chinese Americans rarely eat raw vegetables.	a. Recommend a separate trip to a non-Asian supermarket to buy brown rice b. Congratulate them on eating lots of vegetables c. Congratulate them on eating rice at every meal
10. Southeast Asian mothers calculate age based on the lunar calendar which is based on the different phases of the moon. Reported age can be higher by as much as 2 years, and this may make the child appear to be underweight.	a. Instead of asking mother for baby's age, use baby's birth certificate or chart notes to get date of birth b. Explain to mothers that there is no scientific basis for the lunar calendar. c. Explain baby's growth chart and offer it to Mom for monitoring on the refrigerator door
11. The Chinese believe that the number 4 is bad luck. The Mandarin word for 4 sounds like death. Every week Connecticut casinos send 100 buses to Boston and NYC to transport Chinese Americans to casinos. None of the buses have seats with the number 4. However, the number 8 is considered a lucky number.	a. Offer 4 true/false statements to convince them that the number 4 does not bring bad luck b. Number the statements without using the number 4—1,2,3,5,6,7,8,9 c. Offer 8 true/false statements
12. The Filipino Department of Health has approved garlic for blood cholesterol, ampalaya (bitter melon) for diabetes, and sambong herb for blood pressure.	a. Reinforce benefits of garlic, ampalaya, sambong herb b. Offer taste testing of heart healthy garlic, ampalaya, sambong herb dishes c. Do not mention garlic, ampalaya, or sambong herb because there are no scientific data on these foods.
13. Filipinos have a genetic inability to process large amounts of sodium, showing higher rates of preeclampsia, gestational diabetes, low birth weight babies	Share a. Lists of prohibited high-sodium foods b. Taste testing, recipes, and recommend high-potassium foods for breakfast, lunch, dinner c. Share lists of food-herb pairings as alternatives to monosodium glutamate

Activity--Nutrition Program Planning with Asian Americans

You have secured a consultancy with the local Chinese Cultural Association to celebrate Asian American Heritage Month in May.

Name 10 potential co-sponsors of the planning committee

To the following list of 30-minute interactive learning experiences, add 2 traditional Asian recreational activities which are adapted to team nutrition learning experiences:

Supermarket tour
Ethnic grocery tour
Virtual restaurant tour
Nutrition Bingo
Nutrition Scattegories
Nutrition Jeopardy
Recipe Contest
True/false questions
Digital Nutrition Scavenger Hunt
Analyzing Food Labels
1.

2.

Activity--Finding Asian American Co-sponsors

To the following list of potential Asian American Co-sponsors in South Florida, add two additional Asian American group, and include its address, and email. Search by using descriptors with the name of one of the 50 Asian countries, or the religions--Sikhism, Hinduism, or Buddhism.

Instructions: The first person to add two Asian organizations and their addresses gets a prize.

Potential Asian American Co-Sponsors in South Florida
Coral Springs Chinese Cultural Association, 8343 W. Atlantic Blvd., Coral Springs, FL 33071
Philippine Nurses Association of South Florida, Inc 9500 SW 128 St Miami FL 33176
Morikami Museum and Japanese Gardens, Delray Beach--festivals, tea ceremonies, Ikebana floral arrangement classes, exhibitions
Association of Indians in America, 2298 NW 56th Street, Boca Raton, FL-33496
Asian Pacific American Bar Association of South Florida, 1525 Pennsylvania Ave, Miami, FL 33139
Bangladesh American Chamber of Commerce Florida, 2716 NE 27th Circle, Boca Raton, FL 33431
Bengali Association of South Florida, PO Box 550076, Davie, Florida 33355
Florida China Association, Inc., P.O. Box 226647. Miami, FL 33222-6647
Florida-China Chamber of Commerce, 7200 NW 19th Street, Suite 302, Miami, FL 33126
Hong Kong Association of Florida, Two Biscayne Boulevard Suite 1900, Miami, FL 33131
South Florida Tamil Sangam, 761 SW 190th Av, Pembroke Pines, FL 33029
Taiwanese Chamber of Commerce of Miami, tccmmiami@gmail.com
Asian American Federation of Florida, 659 NE 125th Street, North Miami, FL
Korean American Chamber of Commerce, 525 NW 27th St Miami, FL 33127
Chinese Baptist Church, 6605 SW 88th St, Miami, FL
Miami Vineyard Church 12725 SW 122nd Ave, Miami, FL 33186
Korean Presbyterian Church of Miami
Korean American United Methodist Church of South Florida
Consulate General of Japan, 80 SW 8th St Ste 3200, Miami. (305) 530-9090 www.miami.us.emb-japan.go.jp
Consulate of Thailand in Miami, 2199 Ponce de Leon Blvd., Suite 301. Coral Gables, FL 33134. (305) 445-7577 thaiconsulatemiami@hotmail.com
Honorary Consul General of South Korea, One S.E. Third Ave., 27th floor, Miami, Florida, 33131.

What Would Not Work? For each the following Native American health and cultural norms, choose the inappropriate program feature in a 6-session church weight loss program?

Native American Norm	Program Feature
1.Cultural tolerance for obesity	a. Offer visuals of normal organs in an overweight body b. Share years of life lost due to excess body weight* c. Share a Native American weight loss testimonial
2.Harmony with nature valued	a. Share the top 10 natural foods that can be used to lower blood pressure, cholesterol, sugar b. Recommend Native dishes can reverse nutrition conditions (succotash—beans, corn, squash) c. Warn against using harmful herbs
3.Mixed blood may be respected (Cherokee) or dishonored (Seminole)	a. Link the 50% Rule in portion sizes and frequency to the concept of mixed blood with Cherokee groups b. Do not link 50% Rule to the concept of mixed blood among the Seminole c. Recommend the 50% Rule to Seminole and Cherokee groups
4.Higher unemployment rates	a. Recommend top 10 most nutritious, cheapest foods b. Recommend where to buy the most nutritious, cheapest foods c. Recommend Aldi for lower food prices
5.50% high school dropout rate, compared to 30% nationally	a. Use more white space and visuals, appropriate reading level in flyer, brochures, PowerPoint slides b. Use any Internet document for Native Americans c. Pretest all educational materials
6.The 2014 Native infant mortality rate was 1.6 times higher than the rate for non-Hispanic Whites. Native mothers were 2.5 as likely to receive late or no prenatal care as compared to non-Hispanic White mothers (Centers for Disease Control and Prevention, 2015.	a. Alert them to their higher IMR and share pregnancy weight gain grid b. Target high school girls and boys, pregnant women for nutrition education c. Recommend that pregnant Moms take home the Prenatal Weight Gain Grid during the last trimester
7.The Native adult alcohol mortality rate is five times higher than Whites. The prevalence of Native Fetal Alcohol Syndrome FAS is 33 times higher than Whites. Although Native Americans represent 1% of the population, they have 25% of all FAS babies (8000/y).	a. Teach Refusal Skills to male and female children, teens, adults b. Share alcohol content of foods and over-the-counter medications c. Work with city and tribal councils to ban the sale of alcohol in liquor stores
8.Higher exposure to environmental toxins on Indian Reservations (arsenic and uranium linked to higher cancer rates on Navajo reservations)	Schedule a session a. Less Food Toxins, More Real Foods in My Body! b. More Natural Foods for My Body Today! c. Form an alliance with Native activists to take legal action against the Bureau of Indian Affairs for environmental dumping on Native land

*Years of life lost among overweight persons has been shown to be 3.3 years. For obese and severely obese persons, the number of years of life lost was predicted to be 5.6-7.6 years for men, and 8.1-10.3 years for women aged 20-29 years (Lung, Jan, Tan et al., 2019).

<u>Activity</u>--Nutrition Program Planning with Native Americans

November is Native American Heritage Month. You have approached and secured the co-sponsorship of the largest local Native American newspaper to launch a nutrition program with Native Americans. The newspaper is hoping to improve visibility in the community and to boost declining subscriptions. Identify the Native group at your current or a previous zip code by visiting: 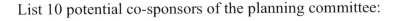 https://native-land.ca/

List 10 potential co-sponsors of the planning committee:

-

-

-

-

-

Identify two Native American traditional recreational activities of that Native American group, and adapt them to team nutrition learning experiences.

Native group's recreational activity—to play….

Seminole nutrition pow wow—To play Seminole nutrition pow wow, after answering a nutrition question correctly, the learner dances for 1 minute with a video of powwow dances, in teams. The winning team has the most dancers.

Supermarket tour
Ethnic grocery tour
Virtual restaurant tour
Nutrition Bingo
Nutrition Scattegories
Nutrition Jeopardy
Recipe Contest
True/False questions
Nutrition Scavenger Hunt
Food Label Comparison
1.
2.

Adapting the Native American Medicine Wheel to a Nutrition Wheel

Identify the Native American Medicine wheel for the local Native group, and convert it to teaching tool for the weight loss program for local Native Americans. Identify the local Native American group from their zip at: https://native-land.ca/

Needs Assessment data indicate:
-Obesity, hypertension, alcoholism, fetal alcohol syndrome, infant mortality, and diabetes and amputation rates which are higher than the national average.
-Cultural tolerance to obesity.
-Poverty rates are three times higher than the national average.

List 4 nutrition topics that you will cover.
-
-
-
-

Original Medicine Wheel   Nutrition Wheel

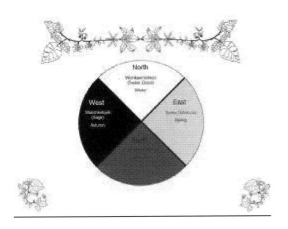

Activity—Indian Talking Stick

The purpose of this classroom activity is to experience the principles of the Indian Talking Stick.

To Make an Indian Talking Stick

You'll need:
-an empty cardboard roll of wrapping paper
-20 dried beans
-tape to seal the roll at both ends,
-a feather which you will attach to the roll.

Seal one end of the cardboard roll with thick paper. Secure the paper with tape.
Pour dried beans in the roll.
Secure the other end of the roll with thick paper.
Attach the feather with clear tape.

The feather is a reminder to take things lightly and to trod lightly on the earth.

Group Discussion--Using the Indian Talking Stick

The purpose of the Group Discussion is to describe strategies for eating more fruit and vegetables while using the Talking Stick. The Stick is given to the person who speaks. As long as the person is speaking, the person holds the Stick. When the person is finished speaking, the person passes the Stick to the next person who will speak.

Each person who holds the Indian Talking Stick:

1. States their name and gives the name of the last person who spoke, and summarizes what the last speaker said.

2. Then the speaker describes how many servings of fruits and vegetables they had yesterday; and says that "tomorrow, I plan to _____ (describe what you will do differently) to ensure that I have one extra serving of fruits or vegetables".

<u>After Action Review</u>
At the end of the activity, allow each person to describe one strength and weakness of using the Indian Talking Stick to increase fruit and vegetable intake.

How could the Indian Talking Stick be adapted for use in a Weight Loss support group among non-Native Americans?

Planning the Anti-Fetal Alcohol Syndrome Prevention among Native Americans

In cooperation with the local Native tribal council, you are planning the Anti Fetal Alcohol Syndrome Prevention among Native Americans.

Answer the following questions:
1. The title for the following list is: ___
        -Seminole women who have FAS babies
        -nurse from Seminole clinic
        -representative from county mental health association
        -representative from county Cooperative Extension
        -Seminole church women who have FAS babies
        -first-time pregnant women
        -Seminole tribal leaders

a. Potential Members of the Planning Committee to Reduce Seminole Fetal Alcohol Syndrome
b. Potential speakers for nutrition sessions
c. Memory jogger titles

2. The nutritionist, community members, and Native tribal council members are planning the anti-Fetal Alcohol Syndrome program. The laundromat, clinics, dental offices, beauty shops, barbershops, convenience stores, corner stores, pharmacies, childcare centers, community centers, gas stations, nail salons, and social media sites represent

a. settings to market the flyer for the FAS program.
b. places to host the 1-hour sessions.
c. settings where clients can make memory joggers.

3. In cooperation with the Native tribal council, an anti-Fetal Alcohol Syndrome program is being planned. Which of the following 30-minute experiences is inappropriate for helping Seminole boys and girls, men and women to prevent FAS?

a. Alcohol Jeopardy; and Alcohol Bingo
b. Alcohol stickball--a Native American team sport which predated lacrosse. To adapt stickball to a learning experience, create two teams, the team which answers alternate questions correctly moves closer to the goal.
c. Role play of Refusal Skills; and an interview with a peer educator—a Mom with a FAS baby or child
d. 4 True/False statements in a Medicine Wheel, followed by a virtual tour of a pharmacy's alcohol-containing over-the-counter medications
e. a 40-minute lecture on Alcohol During Pregnancy

Nutrition Program Planning with Native Hawaiian and Pacific Islanders

What Would Not Work? For each the following Native Hawaiian and Pacific Islander health and nutrition norms, indicate the inappropriate program feature in a 6-session church weight loss program? 20% of Tongans live in Utah; 50% of Samoans, 80% of Fijians live in CA

Native Hawaiian and Pacific Islander Norms	Program Feature
1. Health data are sparse.	a. Consult religious leaders to identify major causes of morbidity, mortality b. Focus on superfoods and the link between food and disease c. Call local physicians in clinics to get health data
2. Cosmic harmony, and Lokahi (equilibrium in all life forces) valued.	a. Incorporate cosmic harmony/lokahi in how foods strengthen the body b. Do not mention cosmic harmony/lokahi because there are no scientific data to support them c. Incorporate the goal of cosmic harmony/lokahi for health indicators—blood pressure, blood sugar
3. Matriarchal society—mothers are influential family members	Target a. mothers for nutrition education b. grandmothers for nutrition education c. boys and men for nutrition education
4. Folk stories, talk story or storytelling	a. Share nutrition success stories with storytellers so that they can incorporate them into talk story b. Invite local storytellers to perform in the nutrition program c. Use mainland folk stories (Johnny Appleseed)
5. Simultaneous overnutrition and undernutrition in the Western Pacific--11.6 million children stunted, and 4.7 million underweight; 60% adolescents are overweight, adult obesity exceeds 50% in many countries (World Health Organization, 2015).	Target a. schools for nutrition education b. seniors for nutrition education c. wait until adolescents become overweight then provide nutrition education
6. Taro, breadfruit, green bananas are often cooked in coconut milk. Kosraean (Micronesian) "all-star" soup features reef fish, crab, and lobster in a rice and coconut milk base.	a. Recommend the 50% Rule for dishes made with white coconut meat b. Describe the health benefits of clear coconut water c. Warn clients of the cholesterol-raising effect of coconut milk, and recommend abstention

Native Hawaiian and Pacific Islander Norms	Program Feature
7. High prevalence of lactose intolerance, calcium deficiency is common	a. Recommend imported Lactaid and Dairy Ease b. Recommend high-calcium, high-absorption cauliflower, greens, broccoli c. Offer tips on weight-bearing exercise
8. Diabetes prevalence is two and a half times higher in Native Hawaiians, five times higher in Guam compared to the mainland	a. Schedule a session: Let's Fight Diabetes with Foods! b. Host a Sugar Shockers guessing experience c. Distribute a 1-page Sugar Shockers handout
9. Peanuts and macadamias are favorites	a. Recommend the 50% rule for peanuts, macadamias. b. Schedule a Mindful Eating activity. c. Recommend buying peanuts in the shell; a small peanut container; a timer to increase time to finish eating.
10. When presented in a traditional Kosrean (Micronesian) feast, the number of breadfruit pieces must be an odd number such as: 3, 5, or 7. However, for healing, the number of leaves musts be four or eight leaf (Leeling, 2011).	In the Nutrition and Healing session, a. Offer 4 true/false statementsfor b. Offer 8 true/false statements c. Offer an odd number of true/false statements

Leeling D. Traditional food dishes of Micronesia. 2011. http://danaleeling.blogspot.com/2011/10/traditional-food-dishes-of-micronesia.html. Accessed July 31, 2019.

Activity--Identifying and Managing Hawaiian Comfort Foods

1. Haupia: coconut pudding (coconut milk, sugar)
2. Shave ice: crushed ice flavored with sweet colored artificially flavored syrup
3. Kalua pig: pork, spices covered with banana leaves and steamed in hot rocks in an underground oven
4. Laulau: steamed fish and pork wrapped in taro and ti leaves
5. Loco moco: hamburger patty topped with fried eggs and gravy
6. Lomilomi salmon: raw, salted salmon with diced tomatoes and onions
7. Malasada: hole-less donut deep fried and coated with sugar
8. Manapua: meat-filled bun, steamed or baked
9. Mochi: Japanese rice cake made of glutinous rice
10. Plate lunch: 2 scoops of white rice, one scoop of macaroni salad, and a hamburger or fried egg
11. Poi: mashed taro (starchy root tuber like boniato)
12. Poke: seasoned raw fish salad
13. Furikake: sesame, salty seaweed sprinkled over anything
14. Arare rice crackers: rice flour, salty
15. Taro rolls: wheat flour and ground taro
16. Taro frozen yogurt (frozen yogurt, sugar, taro)

a. Identify 3 red light foods.
b. Offer one dietary recommendation which Hawaiians could use to reduce the harmful effects of each red light food. Include a recommendation which includes fluids.

RED LIGHT FOOD	RECOMMENDATION WHICH COULD REDUCE THE HARMFUL EFFECTS OF THE RED LIGHT FOOD
1.	i. ii.
2.	i. ii.
3.	i. ii.

Chapter 15

Adapting Nutrition Educational Media to be More Culturally Sensitive

<u>MyPlate Filipino Americans</u>

Review MyPlate.gov for the Filipino version of MyPlate.

How useful is the Filipino MyPlate in a 5-A-Day program for the local Filipino Nurses' Association?
VERY USEFUL/USEFUL/NOT THAT USEFUL

1. Describe two ways that you would use or adapt the Filipino MyPlate for a nutrition program with the local Filipino Nurses' Association.
a.

b.

2. Describe 3 Filipino memory joggers that would be culturally sensitive for the 6-session nutrition program for the local Filipino Nurses' Association.
a.

b.

c.

<u>Adapting the reading level of nutrition education materials</u>
Use the SMOG readability guidelines to assess the reading level of the document *Making the Most of The Food Dollar.* This topic is important to non-Whites, many of whom have lower health literacy levels than Whites. White and non-White Americans often cite the high cost of healthy foods as an obstacle to eating right. However, the topic is particularly valuable to non-Whites who earn 30% less than Whites.

Using the SMOG guidelines in Chapter 15, answer the questions at the end of the document.

Making the Most of Your Supermarket Food Dollar

Plan Ahead

● Plan meals before shopping. Select foods daily from each of these food groups: vegetable-fruit,

bread-cereal, milk-cheese and meat-poultry.

● Fix meals at home to save money.

● Make a shopping list of the foods you need. This lessens the chance of buying extras on impulse.

- Look for specials and coupons in the newspaper ads and magazines. Remember, they save you money only if they are for products you need and normally buy.

- Avoid shopping when you are hungry, tired or in a hurry.

Save at the Store

- Use the "unit price" (price per ounce, pound, or pint) to compare the cost of different brands and package sizes. Many stores show the unit price on the shelf.

- Use open dating information ("sell by" dates and "best if used by" information) to help select the freshest foods.

- Compare ingredient lists and nutrition labels on packaged foods to get the most nutrition for your food dollar.

- Try store brands and generics. They are usually less costly then name brands. They are just as nutritious, too. Buy the "large economy" size only if you have space to store it conveniently and you can use it before part of it spoils. Prevent waste. Avoid over-buying of perishable foods. Compare the cost, quality and preparation time of convenience foods with those you make from scratch. Some convenience foods are bargains. Others, such as frozen combination dishes and ready-to-eat bakery products, can often cost more per serving than similar foods prepared at home. Be flexible. Take advantage of good buys you find at the store. Be ready to substitute one food for another within the following food groups.

Vegetable and Fruit Group

Consider costs per serving of fresh, frozen, and canned fruits and vegetables to find the best buy. Fresh fruits and vegetables are better buys when they are in season than at other times. Plain frozen vegetables are often better buys than those with butter or sauce. Add seasoning yourself to save money.

Bread and Cereal Group

Count on breads, cereals, pasta and other grain products to get more variety in your meals at a low cost. Cereals you cook yourself cost less than instant and ready-to-eat cereals. Regular rice costs less than instant, quick-cooking varieties and seasoned rice mixes. Day-old breads and baked goods may be available at bargain price.

Milk and Cheese Group

Look for less expensive forms of milk-usually fluid skim milk and nonfat dry milk. Large containers (a gallon of fluid milk or a big box of nonfat dry milk) are often the most economical. Check the unit price to be sure. You can use yogurt, cheese and other milk products to replace some of the milk in your diet, although milk provides calcium at lower cost.

Meat, Poultry, Fish and Beans Group

Think of cost per serving, not cost per pound, when buying meat, poultry and fish. After cooking, you can get three 3-ounce servings of lean meat per pound from an item with little or no fat or bone, like round steak. On the other hand, you can get only one serving of lean meat per pound from an item with a greater amount of bone, gristle and fat, like spareribs. Some of the best buys are chicken, turkey; beef liver, ground beef and pork shoulder. Lean meat from a lower cost cut is as nutritious as lean meat from a higher cost cut. For example, round steak, trimmed of fat, is as nutritious as a porterhouse steak, trimmed of fat. If you have enough freezer space, you can buy meats on sale and store them for future use. Eggs, dry beans, dry peas and peanut butter are protein sources, too. Use them for economy and variety.

Fats, Sweets and Alcohol Group

Keep in mind that fats, sweets and alcoholic beverages provide calories but   little or no nutrients for the money spent. These "extras" can add variety to your meals but you should not replace more nutritious foods in your diet.

Questions:

1. Number of sentences: _____

2. Sentence #____ is the first sentence of the middle 10 sentences.

3. Sentence #____ is the last sentence of the middle 10 sentences.

4. Sentence # ___ is the first sentence of the last 10 sentences.

5. Total # of polysyllabic words in the first 10 sentences=

6. Total # of polysyllabic words in the middle 10 sentences=

7. Total # of polysyllabic words in the last 10 sentences=

8. Total # of polysyllabic sentences in the document=

9. Using the SMOG Conversion table, the reading level of this document: _____

Revise the last 7 sentences so that they do not contain any polysyllabic words.

Original Sentence	Revised Sentence

Place three visuals of specific foods that you would use to reinforce the main messages in this document. At least one visual should include price comparisons.
Include a call to action with each visual as a call to action. The caption should contain no polysyllabic words.

1.

2.

3.

<u>Improving the Reading Level of Nutrition Education Materials for Central Americans</u>
According to a 2015 Academy of Nutrition and Dietetics survey of health professionals with experience in Central America, populations in developing areas of this region lack basic knowledge of biology and physiology. This document *Explaining Organ Functions (Central Americans)* was developed to discuss basic health concepts and then explain how nutrition affects our bodies is a good strategy.

Determine the reading level of the document by answering the following questions:

1. Number of sentences: _____

2. Sentence #_____ is the first sentence of the middle 10 sentences.

3. Sentence #_____ is the last sentence of the middle 10 sentences.

4. Sentence #_____ is the first sentence of the last 10 sentences.

5. Total # of polysyllabic words in the first 10 sentences=

6. Total # of polysyllabic words in the middle 10 sentences=

7. Total # of polysyllabic words in the last 10 sentences=

8. Total # of sentences=

9. From the SMOG Conversion table, the reading level of this document: _____

Revise the last 10 sentences so that they contain no polysyllabic words.

Original Sentence	Revised Sentence

Place three visuals of specific foods that you would use to reinforce the main messages in this document. At least one visual should include price comparisons.
Include a call to action with each visual. The caption should contain no polysyllabic words.

1.

2.

3.

Explaining Organ Functions (Central Americans)

<u>Using Literacy Guidelines for Central America</u>
According to a 2015 Academy of Nutrition and Dietetics survey of health professionals with experience in Central America, populations in developing areas of this region lack basic knowledge of biology and physiology. Beginning with a discussion of basic health concepts and then explaining how nutrition affects our bodies is a good strategy.

Review this section of the document *Explaining Organ Functions (Central Americans)* which is designed for nutrition professionals. Identify three strengths and weaknesses.

3 Strengths:
1.
2.
3.

3 Weaknesses
1.
2.
3.

Explaining Organ Functions (Central Americans)

- Lungs: provide oxygen to blood
- Heart: circulates blood throughout the body
- Stomach: helps digest food
- Intestines: absorb nutrients from food
- Liver: removes toxins from blood and processes nutrients from food
- Kidneys: filter blood of waste and extra fluid

Explaining Nutrition

Nutrition is how food affects the health of the body. Food is essential—it provides vital nutrients for survival, and helps the body function and stay healthy. Food is comprised of macronutrients including protein, carbohydrate and fat that not only offer calories to fuel the body and give it energy but play specific roles in maintaining health. Food also supplies micronutrients (vitamins and minerals) and phytochemicals that don't provide calories but serve a variety of critical functions to ensure the body operates optimally.

Explaining Macronutrients: Protein, Carbohydrate and Fat

Protein: Found in beef, pork, chicken, game and wild meats, fish and seafood, eggs, soybeans and other legumes included in traditional Central America cuisine, protein provides the body with amino acids. Amino acids are the building blocks of proteins which are needed for growth, development, and repair and maintenance of body tissues. Protein provides structure to muscle and bone, repairs tissues when damaged and helps immune cells fight inflammation and infection.

Carbohydrates: The main role of a carbohydrate is to provide energy and fuel the body the same way gasoline fuels a car. Foods such as corn, chayote, beans, plantains, rice, tortilla, potatoes and other root vegetables such as yucca, bread and fruit deliver sugars or starches that provide carbohydrates for energy.

Energy allows the body to do daily activities as simple as walking and talking and as complex as running and moving heavy objects. Fuel is needed for growth, which makes sufficient fuel especially important for growing children and pregnant women. Even at rest, the body needs calories to perform vital functions such as maintaining body temperature, keeping the heart beating and digesting food.

Fat: Dietary fat, which is found in oils, coconut, nuts, milk, cheese, meat, poultry and fish, provides structure to cells and cushions membranes to help prevent damage. Oils and fats are also essential for absorbing fat-soluble vitamins including vitamin A, a nutrient important for healthy eyes and lungs.

Explaining Micronutrients: Vitamins and Minerals

Vitamins and minerals are food components that help support overall health and play important roles in cell metabolism and neurological functions.

Vitamins aid in energy production, wound healing, bone formation, immunity, and eye and skin health.

Minerals help maintain cardiovascular health and provide structure to the skeleton.

Consuming a balanced diet including fruits, vegetables, dairy, protein foods and whole or enriched grains helps ensure the body has plenty of nutrients to use. Providing a few examples of specific micronutrient functions can enhance the effectiveness of nutrition education:

- **Vitamin A** helps the eyes to see
- **Calcium and magnesium** help muscles and blood vessels relax, preventing cramps and high blood pressure
- **Vitamin C** helps wounds heal and the body's ability to fight off germs
- **Iron** helps the blood transport oxygen throughout the body and prevents anemia

Explaining the Concept of Nutrients as Building Blocks

Building blocks include protein for growing babies in utero, for child and adolescent growth, and for repairing damaged skin, blood, and other body parts in adults who aren't growing. Some parts of the body are replaced regularly, like blood and skin, so even adults are building new body parts regularly. Calcium is also a building block for building bones. Iron is a building block for blood. Since blood cells only last a few months, the body constantly needs more iron and protein to make new blood.

Using Metaphors to Explain Nutrition

According to registered dietitian nutritionists with experience teaching nutrition in developing areas of Central America, metaphors and simple concepts are useful in teaching basic nutrition. An example of this could be conveying foods rich in carbohydrate as "go" foods, protein-rich foods as "grow" foods and colorful produce as "glow" foods. Health educators should emphasize that good nutrition requires eating at least one serving of these three types of food at each meal: 〽

Foods	Simple Concept of Function
Carbohydrate-rich foods	Fuel
Protein-rich foods	Building blocks
Fruits and Vegetables	Helpers and protectors

From: https://www.eatrightpro.org/practice/practice-resources/international-nutrition-pilot-project/how-to-explain-basic-nutrition-concepts

<u>Activity--Adapting True/False Statements</u>
1. Does Figure A or B contain True/False statements which are more user-friendly to multiethnic Black barbershop patrons? Offer a rationale for your choice.

Figure A
True/False Statements
What's Your Prostate Cancer IQ?

TRUE/ FALSE/ Don't Know

1.____ **African-American** men and White men have the same risk of dying from prostate cancer.

2.____ The most **effective** way to reduce prostate cancer risk in **African-American** men over the age of 50 is to eat more fruits and **vegetables**.

3.____ **African-American** men have 13% more of the male sex hormone testosterone than White men.

4.____ Cooked tomatoes, pink grapefruit, pink guava and watermelon can improve the health of the prostate gland.

5.____ **African-American** men have the highest death rate from prostate cancer in the world.

Figure B
True/False Statements
What's Your Prostate Cancer IQ?

TRUE/ FALSE/ Don't Know

1.____ Black and White men have the same risk of dying from prostate cancer.

2.____ The best way to reduce prostate cancer risk in Black men over the age of 50 is to eat more fruits and veggies.

3.____ Black men have 13% more of the male sex hormone testosterone than white men.

4.____ Cooked tomatoes, pink grapefruit, pink guava and watermelon can improve the health of the prostate gland.

5.____ Black men have the highest death rate from prostate cancer in the world.

Guidelines for Using Existing Nutrition Educating Materials with Clients

The table below was extracted from the American Diabetes Association's "Managing Diabetes Among Mexican Americans", 2010.

Fats	Carbohydrate	Alternative Sweeteners	Sodium
-Reduce oil used in preparing soups to <1 tsp. -Prepare frijoles cocidos (boiled beans) instead of frijoles refritos (refried beans). -Grill meats and tortillas instead of frying them. -Chill and skim fat off broth when making caldos (soups). -Use low-fat milk instead of whole milk and cream. -Avoid high-fat cheeses using part-skim milk queso fresco instead. -Restrict chorizo (sausage) and menudo (tripe soup) to special occasions. -Drain fat from fried chorizo, and trim visible fat from meats.	-Use corn tortillas instead of flour tortillas. -Make tortillas from scratch using whole-wheat flour and appropriate type of margarine. -Include beans daily to maintain high levels of soluble dietary fiber consumption. -Increase intake of fresh fruits and vegetables. -Drink water or diet soda instead of sweetened soft drinks. If diabetes is controlled and body weight is reasonable, occasionally incorporate sweets, such as pan dulce. -Account for all calories in the total mean plan. Use no added sugar in licuados and aguas frescas.	-Sweetened carbonated soft drinks need to be replaced with water and diet sodas. -Use artificial sweeteners in coffee and atole (hot beverage thickened with cornstarch).	-Taste food before using salt. -Minimize consumption of salty snack foods, such as chips, chicharrones (fried pork rinds), and dips. Instead of salt, use lemon in beer or on fruits such as melon. -Add flavor to foods using onion, garlic, cumin, oregano, cilantro, and other spices.

Identify one statement with which you disagree:

Write the revised version of the statement:

Background information:
Although many health-related organizations like the American Diabetes Association, the Academy of Nutrition and Dietetics, and the American Medical Association recommend sugar substitutes for persons with diabetes, many nutrition advocacy organizations believe that the risks are greater than the benefits because they change DNA structure and cause cancer. No long-term studies have ever been done on the safety for humans.

RDN OBSTACLES TO BUILDING RAPPORT

RDN STATEMENTS	CLIENT'S UNSPOKEN RESPONSE/BARRIER	MORE APPROPRIATE STATEMENTS:
1."Hi" with a big smile, extending a hand to Mr. Cox, a Trinidadian American whose blood cholesterol is high.	"I wish she was Trinidadian like me".	1."Good morning Mr. Cox. I am Ms. Allen, the registered dietitian nutritionist here. Please have a seat. How can I help you today?" 2."I'm not as ……………. as I'd like to be about Trinidadian cuisine. How often do you get to eat Trinidadian foods?"
2."You guys will really benefit from this program" to a group of older Seminole tribal leaders who are being asked to fund a 6-session Weight Loss program. (Seminoles call themselves "The Unconquered" because they are the only Native American tribe that did not surrender to the White man over three wars).	"She's so unprofessional!".	1."Gentlemen, we have designed this program specifically for Seminoles. The reading level of all educational materials is appropriate—at …….. grade level to make them easy to read and understand. For the Unconquered, we will focus on strategies to c……………. temptation. Since many of our clients respond well to success stories, we will also showcase local ………….. who have successfully lost weight and kept it off".
"Do you understand?"	I wish I knew what these foods taste like, how much they cost, and where to find them. A closed-ended question may result in a "Yes" or "No" response. This does not lead to a dialogue between RDN and client.	"Could you list three of the recommended ……. that you would be willing to try?"

Overcoming Barriers to Participation and Retention in Nutrition Programs

For each of the following scenarios, propose one strategy to improve nutrient intake among older Americans

Low Access Scenario to the Older Americans Act OAA (Meals on Wheels, congregate meals)	Strategies
1.*Only 244 of 500 Native American tribes are served by the OAA. The Native American poverty rate is three times higher than Whites.	
2.*The OAA Nutrition Program reaches less than 33% of eligible older adults.	
3.*Less than 5% of eligible older Americans receive Meals-On-Wheels.	
4.*On average, older Americans who participate in home-delivered or congregate receive less than three meals per week.	
5.The Senior Farmers' Market Nutrition Program offers fresh, nutritious, locally grown fruits, vegetables, herbs, and honey from farmers' markets, roadside stands, and community-supported agriculture programs. In 2010, benefits ranged from $20 per year to $50 per year among 844,999 older adults. There 46 million Americans who are over 60 years of age, with a poverty rate of 15%. https://us.sagepub.com/sites/default/files/upm-binaries/54297_Chapter_10.pdf	

*Zhu H, An R. Impact of home-delivered meal programs on diet and nutrition among older adults: A review. Nutrition and Health. 2013 Apr;22(2):89–103.

Case Study—Mr. Lin's Level of Rapport with the RDN

Mr. Chu Lin is a Chinese-American has been diagnosed with high blood cholesterol (280 mg/dl versus the recommended 200 mg/dl). He has been referred to the registered dietitian nutritionist by his physician and has arrived at the consultation with his granddaughter who speaks English.

OBSTACLE	STRATEGY
1.Mr. Lin, who eats Chinese foods exclusively enters the hospital RDN's office, looks around briefly, and sees a MyPlate poster of mainstream American foods. The only recognizable food to him is broccoli.	
2.He enters the dietitian's office. He brought his bilingual granddaughter along to serve as interpreter because he does not speak English.	
3.Mr. Lin is in his sixties and notices that the dietitian appears to be in her 30s. She seems so young to him.	
4.He is conservative in his manner and dress, notices that the dietitian is wearing a fuchsia blouse. The fuchsia seems a bit loud to him. He noticed her bright red lipstick, and immediately thought that it looked as if she had swallowed a rat. He looks at her ID, hoping to find out if she is really the dietitian but he does not read English.	
5.As Mr. Lin enters the office, the dietitian sits at the round table. She does not offer any gestures on where he should sit. He sits as far away as possible from the loud fuchsia blouse and the bright red lipstick.	
6."Hi Chu. I'm Tracy. How are you doing?" says the dietitian, without acknowledging his granddaughter's presence.	
7.Mr. Lin has no health insurance and is wondering how much this session will cost. He decides against making that inquiry now.	

If you were Mr. Lin, would you return for the follow-up visit?

Recovering from a Cross-Cultural Oops!

WHAT HAPPENED	CONSEQUENCES	THE CULTURALLY COMPETENT APPROACH
RDN to a Turkish American woman: "How do you celebrate Christmas?"	Mrs Fattah feels a sense of disconnect with the RDN. (Turkey is a predominantly Muslim country).	"Which holidays do you .... in Turkey"
RDN congratulates a Hmong mother on her baby and says "She's beautiful"	The Hmong mother turns red in fear. The Hmong believe that good-looking infants attract evil spirits that will inhabit the infant.	"I'm so .... to see both of you!"
RDN recommends that during the fasting season of Ramadan, a Muslim client who has been diagnosed with diabetes should continue to eat and drink water in order to stabilize blood sugar levels.	Despite the RDN's recommendations, client chooses to uphold Islamic law which forbids water and food from dusk till dawn. Hypoglycemia results and she passes out at work.	"During Ramadan, it's more important than usual to take your diabetes medicine on time and at the .... dosage". You might want to mention this to your physician to find out about the best medication dosage during ....
A flyer for an Osteoporosis program includes a snowboard shape of Asian flags.	Older Asian Americans are offended because they interpret the snowboard as a phallic symbol (represents a penis). No one attends the program.	Pretest .... educational materials and flyers with the target population.
Sharing the top 10 low-fat dairy sources of calcium with Blacks or Asians during the first diabetes support group session.	Because many Blacks and Asians are lactose intolerant, they experience abdominal discomfort and diarrhea when they eat dairy products. They do not feel that this information is useful, reducing their intention of returning to future sessions.	Explore "What's making it .... for them to eat calcium-rich non-dairy foods?"

Case Study—Improving attendance and retention of a hospital diabetes support group

As the new registered dietitian nutritionist at ABC General Hospital, you have inherited a free diabetes support group which meets on Tuesdays 3 pm. Attendance began with eight clients. Following national trends where the number of original participants drops by half midway through the program, halfway through the program, attendance dropped to four participants.

Needs assessment data reveal that:
-The city in which the hospital is located is 46.5% White, 25.3% multiethnic Hispanic, and 20.8% multiethnic Black.
-Half of the Blacks are Caribbean Americans. For this quarter, you have decided to target the Caribbean American population for the diabetes support group.
-Their nutrition problems are overweight/obesity, cultural tolerance to overweight/obesity, hypertension, diabetes, hypercholesterolemia, and prostate cancer.

Add one obstacle, strategy and resource to the table below.

OBSTACLES	STRATEGIES	RESOURCES
3 pm meeting time	Change meeting time to ___ pm	Approval from Human Resources for RDN flex time—to work from 12 noon to 8 pm on meeting days
Potential clients are concerned that the sessions will be a lecture	Describe the format of each session in the flyer—10-minute presentation, and then a fun, _____ learning experience-- Caribbean virtual grocery tour, virtual Caribbean restaurant tour; prizes	Guidelines on developing a culturally sensitive lesson plan
No transportation	Church _____	Church approval
Potential clients see no benefit of attending	-Share the program benefits in the flyer— *'Come and find out which Caribbean foods can reverse diabetes'*, -Describe the skills that learners will acquire: a. list strategies to overcome dietary _____ to reversing diabetes; b. how to save 20% on your food bill.	-Internet search for Caribbean _____ for diabetes -Apply the Cross-Cultural Nutrition Checklist to the flyer in order to maximize its cultural sensitivity of the flyer. -Use the guidelines for developing a culturally sensitive flyer.
Clients have not heard of the diabetes support group	a. Distribute flyer in Caribbean barbershops, beauty shops, churches, grocery stores, newspapers, restaurants, the Caribbean radio stations, and the Caribbean _____. b. Co-sponsor a Caribbean Walk-a-thon with the Caribbean consulates.	a. Get flyer approval from barbershops, beauty shops, churches; grocery stores, restaurants; the Jamaican, Bahamian, Barbadian, Trinidadian, St. Lucian consulates. -Place advertisements in Caribbean newspapers, on the Caribbean _____ stations. b. Co-sponsorships with consulates.

Diverse Community Questionnaire

As part of the **journaling assignment**, interns will complete the *Diverse Community Questionnaire*. The *Diverse Community Questionnaire* will expose the intern to the organizations and/or agencies respect to cultural competency, diversity and inclusion (social inclusion) to the community served. Interns will complete the questionnaire and should discuss the findings with the preceptor. *Cultural competency, diversity and inclusion* cross all aspects of practice. **Type in detail the journal answers and submit at the end of the rotation. Answers to the journal questions should be concise and specific to the rotation. Preceptor will sign final journal entries.**

1. Target population

   a. what is the service population's neighborhood/community location?

   (ethnicity, age, race, color, gender, socio-economic status, nationality, citizenship, education, geographic origin, religion, gender orientation)

   b. what is the community's religious/spiritual beliefs and practices?

   c. what are the primary languages of the community?

2. Has the organization and/or agency provided services to this community?

   a. yes, did the organization and/or agency includes the community in developing service(s), policy and procedures and mission statement?

   b. no, does the organization and/or agency plan to include the community in developing service(s), policy and procedures and mission statement?

3. If your organization and/or agency has serviced or currently serves the community, what has the organization and/or agency learned about the community that could be helpful in providing better service?

   a. what feedback has the organization and/or agency received about services?

   b. what can your organization and/or agency do to improve or enhance the services?

c. how does the community being served perceive the organization and/or agency?

d. how does your staff characterize the community being served?

4. What are the structural and cultural barriers to services provided to community?

5. What are the cultural barriers that limit services to a population in the community?

a. what steps could the organization and/or agency take to reduce or eliminate

cultural barriers to services for the community population?

6. How can your organization and/or agency improve or enhance the community's perspective?

7. Does your preceptor or member of the team support an agency by participating on advisory boards and/or committees serving the community?

Analyze the data gathered from the Diversity Questionnaire. Based on the data, explain 'how' the rotation site uses this data to provide care to the patient/client. Give examples of 'how' the information gathered from the Diversity Questionnaire is or could be used by the site.

Source: Dr. Dona Greenwood, Keiser University

Making Oral Presentations

A common mistake among nutrition educators is to attempt to cover too _____ information in the time allotted. It is essential to determine, in advance, what you want the learners to be able to FEEL and DO at the _____ of the presentation. Ideally, learners need to feel more confident about their ability to make dietary changes; and they need to have learned practical skills: list 3 low-fat dairy products, 3 low-sugar high-fiber cereals, 2 heart-healthy fast food options, or 3 heart-healthy snacks.

When you rehearse your presentation, audiotape it, and listen to it for strengths and areas of _____.

Oral presentations should generally be limited to 5-10 major points—each of which should be _____ through examples, nutrition success stories, and interactive learning activities like nutrition soccer. Although the allotted timing of the presentation may vary from 10 to 90 minutes, attention span is usually limited by chronological _____, it rarely exceeds 20 minutes. A 15-year old probably has an attention span of 15 minutes, but a 25-year old still has an attention span of 20 _____. The secret to effective nutrition education is to ADAPT the presentation to the _____ and motivational level of the learners.

INTRODUCTION

To establish credibility with the learners: The nutrition educator should:

1. determine the purpose of the presentation—how the learners will feel (confident, excited) and what they will know at the end of the presentation.
2. make reference to your .... with that topic or group, your professional experience "Over the years I've noticed..."
3. describe what learners will be able to do by the .... of the presentation—Answer their unasked question: What's In It For Me WIIFM?
4. review the .... which will be discussed. First, the relationship between diet and cancer; Second, which high-fiber peas and beans, the best breakfast cereals; Third, how to read food labels for fat and fiber.
5. share a personal .... of how she resolved a personal nutrition challenge. "Years ago, I never used to eat........... but nowadays..."
6. provide a copy of their resume to the person who will .... you prior to the presentation, highlighting your educational credentials, experience and the main take-away point of the presentation. To allow the person who is introducing you to leave out details which could reduce your credibility demonstrates poor preparation.

Refrain from sharing how nervous you are at the beginning of the presentation with the learners. Sharing this information does not make you less nervous. Instead the learners begin to focus on your discomfort. However, they are not in a position to relieve your discomfort. Prepare in advance to manage pre-presentation jiggers.

The BODY of the presentation

This component describes the points which had been mentioned in the introduction but during the body of the presentation they will be described in _____ detail. To maximize the learners' understanding and retention:

1. be sensitive to the learners' responses and ask for _____ when you notice non-verbal cues of confusion ("I'm noticing an expression on your face, what were you thinking?", or discomfort or displeasure ("You seem uncomfortable. What has been said that offends you?") Decide beforehand whether you plan to ignore latecomers or help them find a _____.

2. _____ genuinely to reflect gentleness, approachableness and non-defensiveness

3. make eye contact with _____ people around the room. Looking over the heads of people in the last row creates _____ between the presenter and the learners. The audience assumes the emotions of the speaker. If you are fidgety, unsure or uncomfortable, the learners will inherit your energy. On the other hand, if you practice sufficiently and make corrections, you will soon be able to make your enthusiasm, fun, and confidence spill ……………….. onto the learners. There are really three speeches—the one you mentally rehearse, the one you really give, and the one you wish you had given. Practice!

4. vary the tone and pitch (how high or low the voice is) ………………. to keep learners interested.

5. vary your speed of …………….. to fit the needs of the group. Because we can think and read five times faster than we can speak, it would be a _____ for the nutrition educator to read along with learners from a slide. Use the opportunity to tell a story and _……………… on the important points.

6. Stand as …………...to the learners if possible. Throughout the presentation, circulating among the learners sends a message that you are _____ with them. Standing behind a podium may be helpful to the speaker but it inadvertently creates physical and emotional _____ between the learners and the nutrition educator.

7. To assess the helpfulness of a behavior, ask yourself the question: Does it build a bridge or a …………?

8. If you use note cards, increase the size of the font so that you will look only momentarily at the cards. That way you will be able to make more _____ contact with the learners.

9. invite learners to ask questions …………….. the presentation. If you don't know the answer to the question, simply say "That's a good question. You know, I'm not sure… I'll check on it and let you know. How can I ……………. the information to everyone?"

CONCLUDING THE PRESENTATION

To ensure that you have time for the conclusion, keep _____ of the time. It is more important to sacrifice some of the content so that you will get to the _____. "To conclude, I want to leave you with one more thought about ..." At the beginning of the talk, invite learners to ask questions. For every question that is asked, there are seven other learners who had the same question but _____ not to ask that question. For every written consumer complaint, there are another 99 consumers who did not _____ to communicate their feelings. Summarize the talk with: "To pull all of this together..."

Workshop Presentations

--usually last more than 90 minutes and may consist of a series of presentations which are linked together. It is critical to determine how _____ learners are with workshop activities because this gives the nutrition educator an opportunity to make programmatic _____.

Media Presentations

More than 50% of listeners' interpretation of the message is communicated by the speaker's manner, energy, and level of _____. It is therefore necessary to be slightly _____ animated during radio or television appearances. Before scheduling the segment, be sure to determine:

a. how much _____ will be allotted to your segment. Electronic media run on a strict non-negotiable schedule for advertisements and station identification. Nothing is worse than running out of time and you didn't get to make your main _____.

b. which questions will be asked by the _____

During the media appearance:

1. Keep the message simple and be sure to _____ it. "It's important to eat the right fats in the right amount."

2. Reinforce important points with "The truth of the matter is that..." "Many people think that... but..."

3. Use commercial _____ to ensure that the interviewer asks specific questions.

4. Keep hand gestures to a _____ because it can be distracting to viewers.

5. If you are pushed to focus on a topic for which you are not _____, assertively state "I would rather not discuss that. The main point here is that…"

6. If other panel members interrupt, without verbal or non-verbal expression, assertively state "Please let me finish my point!"

7. Conclude the media appearance with a definitive statement which is related to the _____ such as "It's important to remember that …"

8. Thank the producer and director _____ after the show. Only ask for feedback if you can _____ it.

Before delivering any oral presentation, be sure that you identify your own personal physical stress response, develop a plan and _____ the plan to manage the stress response. For many presenters, the time of greatest anxiety is just _____ the presentation begins. After that, it gets easier as you get fully _____ in the presentation.

Managing Your Pre-Presentation Jitters

1. What are your personal symptoms of nervousness?

A churning stomach, sweaty palms, diarrhea, dry mouth?

2. For your personal symptom, identify two things that you could do to reduce the effect of the symptom (state specific foods or beverages, if applicable):

My anxiety symptom:

To reduce the effect of the symptom, I could:

1.

2.

Symptom: heart racing/increased heart rate

To reduce the effect of the symptom, I could:

i. Make sure not to eat caffeine-containing foods (coffee yogurt or ice cream) or drink caffeine in soda, coffee, energy drinks (Red Bull; or take over-the-counter medications.

ii. Enjoy more chamomile, turmeric, green tea, water; while breathing deeply.

Communicating with Persons who have Hearing Loss

- Speak up, but do not shout. Ask the person if you are speaking loud enough or too
  _____.
- Speak _____--but don't exaggerate your speech so that it becomes distorted.
- Rephrase rather than _____ a misunderstood sentence. If the person is still not
  understanding you, offer to _____ it down.
- If you are giving someone information where details are important, write it down and ask
  them to _____ it to be sure that they understand correctly.
- Decrease background noise by moving away from a crowded area or by turning _____
  the TV or radio.
- Face the listener and make sure that the light is on your _____, not shining in their
  eyes. People with hearing loss, even if they are wearing hearing aids, need to lip-read to
  compensate for the _____ that they miss. Be sure your mouth is not covered by your
  _____, or any obstruction like a toothpick, cigarette, food or gum.
- Get the person's attention _____ you begin speaking. NEVER try to talk to a
  person with hearing loss from another _____.
- Choose the best time to communicate and be patient—people with hearing problems have
  more difficulties when they are tired or _____.

Communicating with Older Adults

For each of the following age-related changes, insert an appropriate communication strategy

CHANGES IN AGING	COMMUNICATION STRATEGY FOR OLDER ADULTS
Decreased visual acuity	
Inability to see blue, green, and violet	
Increased glare	

Getting Better at Making Oral Presentations

The best presenters have a history of preparing and reviewing their presentations. To prepare to answer the question that will occur to you at the end of the presentation:

"How did I do?",

audiotape every presentation. Set up your audio recording system in a way that you cannot begin the presentation without seeing the cue to start recording. If you are using a cell phone to audiotape the presentation, use you cell phone as a reminder and place it on _____ of the pointer or the clicker.

1. As soon as you leave the presentation, _____ to the audiotape.

2. Identify the strengths and weaknesses. Convert each weakness into a TO DO list for your _____ presentation.

Your personal goal is to use learners' feedback to keep getting _____. Over the years, you will be amazed at how much your presentation style improves, with practice and perpetual _____ of the strengths and weaknesses.

One of the best structured ways to become a better public speaker is to join Toastmasters International and give 10 short speeches, receive feedback and become a Toastmaster.

State the address and meeting time of the closest Toastmasters International meeting to your home and university zip code

i. home:

ii. university:

REFERENCES

Dresser, N. *Multicultural Manners: Essential Rules of Etiquette for the 21st Century.* 2005. New York: Wiley.

U.S. Department of Agriculture, Food and Nutrition Service, Office of Policy Support, *Characteristics of Supplemental Nutrition Assistance Program Households: Fiscal Year 2017,* by Kathryn Cronquistand Sarah Lauffer. Project Officer, Jenny Genser. Alexandria, VA, 2019.

ABOUT THE AUTHOR

Since 1991, as an Associate Professor of Nutrition at Florida International University, Dr. Magnus has devoted her research to evaluating nutrition education approaches on prostate cancer in Haitian American, English-speaking Caribbean, and African American barbershops. There she discovered how different ethnic groups had varying preferences in nutrition education. Her research on weight perception among Cuban American mothers in the Women, Infants, and Children program, and Haitian American outpatients generated alarming data on the persistence of weight misperception among non-Whites. Her qualitative research with opinion leaders of 15 ethnic groups and three religions—Christianity, Buddhism, and Islam—distilled the factors which were linked to funded nutrition proposals. As the External Evaluator of a semester-long, university-based weight loss program for five years, she gained valuable insights into the learning and cultural needs of multiethnic Black and Hispanic faculty members, staff, and students; the registered dietitian nutrition, and personal trainers.

She has published extensively on nutrition education—the need for, the effectiveness of different nutrition education approaches among non-Whites, older African American, Jewish American, and Caribbean American adults, multiethnic Black and Hispanic. As a Professor, she has directed or served on the committees of more than 30 Masters theses and PhD dissertations.

She has been an invited speaker to national and state dietetic association meetings of dietitians and nutritionists in Miami, Tampa, Los Angeles, and San Diego; the South Florida District Dental Association of dental hygienists, and dentists (Miami), the American Diabetes Association Florida Affiliate, Inc (Miami), the International Conference of the American Diabetes Association and the University of the West Indies (Jamaica), the Caribbean Association of Nutritionists and Dietitians (the Bahamas, Jamaica), the Canadian Dietetic Association (Ottawa), Caribbean Studies Association (Trinidad and Tobago), the Ministry of Health (Barbados), and Changhi General Hospital (Singapore).

She has taught undergraduate and graduate nutrition courses at 1) the University of the West Indies Distance Learning Nutrition Course broadcast to 154 nutrition and health professionals in 11 Caribbean countries (based in Jamaica); 2) Jamaica's University of Technology Masters' in Public Health Nutrition to students in multiple Caribbean countries; and 3) Jinan University, Guangzhou, China for three years.

As the Public Health Nutritionist at the World Health Organization/Caribbean Food and Nutrition Institute/Pan American Health Organization (PAHO), she provided technical assistance in nutrition to 19 Caribbean countries. In this role, she conducted training in nutrition services, and coordinated the National Food Consumption Survey of Dominica.

In her PAHO consultancies, she led Log Frame planning workshops for nutritionists and dietitians in 19 Caribbean countries; and wrote the National Plan of Action for three Caribbean countries--the Bahamas, Montserrat, and Dominica. As a Consultant to Home Study Educators, she served as Editor of two nutrition books for dental hygienists and dentists.

As the External Examiner of the Dietetics and Nutrition Programme at the University of Technology, Jamaica for eight years, she evaluated the undergraduate curriculum to ensure that it met international standards. As a Fullbright Scholar to Barbados, she documented the prevalence of drug-nutrient interactions among outpatients. She served as Guest Expert on "International Nutrition" Graham Kerr's *The Galloping Gourmet* television program in Toronto, Canada, aired to 13 million viewers worldwide.

As a Jamaican American who has lived in the United States for more than 30 years, she has blended her professional perspective as a nutrition researcher and her perspective as a Jamaican, and the perspectives of Jamaican friends and family members.

Dr. Magnus has travelled to, or worked in nutrition in more than 60 countries.

Made in the USA
Columbia, SC
13 January 2021